LAZY, CRAZY, AND DISGUSTING

LAZY, CRAZY, AND DISGUSTING

Stigma and the Undoing of Global Health

ALEXANDRA BREWIS

AMBER WUTICH

Johns Hopkins University Press | Baltimore

© 2019 Johns Hopkins University Press
All rights reserved. Published 2019
Printed in the United States of America on acid-free paper

Johns Hopkins Paperback edition, 2022
9 8 7 6 5 4 3 2 1

Johns Hopkins University Press
2715 North Charles Street
Baltimore, Maryland 21218-4363
www.press.jhu.edu

The Library of Congress has cataloged the hardcover edition of this book as follows:

Names: Brewis, Alexandra, author. | Wutich, Amber, author.
Title: Lazy, crazy, and disgusting : stigma and the undoing
    of global health / Alexandra Brewis and Amber Wutich.
Description: Baltimore : Johns Hopkins University Press, 2019. |
    Includes bibliographical references and index.
Identifiers: LCCN 2019010086 | ISBN 9781421433356 (hardcover : alk. paper) |
    ISBN 1421433354 (hardcover : alk. paper) | ISBN 9781421433363 (electronic) |
    ISBN 1421433362 (electronic)
Subjects: | MESH: Global Health—ethnology | Social Stigma | Attitude
    to Health | Sanitation | Obesity | Mental Disorders
Classification: LCC RA441 | NLM WA 530.1 | DDC 362.1—dc23
LC record available at https://lccn.loc.gov/2019010086

A catalog record for this book is available from the British Library.

ISBN 978-1-4214-4325-6

Special discounts are available for bulk purchases of this book.
For more information, please contact Special Sales at specialsales@jh.edu.

Contents

Acknowledgments

The argument we build in this book reflects a shared intellectual journey over the past decade, and along the way we have had much help from many colleagues. At the School of Human Evolution and Social Change (SHESC) at Arizona State University (ASU), we are extremely lucky to be part of an incredibly energetic and supportive research team. We particularly thank those who have come willingly on various parts of this adventure with us, collaborating on research and teaching, traveling with us to field sites, working with us on the publications that form the evidence base of parts of this book, providing a sounding board or other vital support at key junctures. A special thanks to those wonderful SHESC colleagues who worked directly with us at ASU on a range of collaborative activities we discuss in this text: Gina Agostini, Melissa Beresford, Russ Bernard, Drew Blasco, Christopher Boone, Meg du Bray, Cinthia Carvajal, Jose Rosales Chavez, Danelle Cooper, Christine DeMyers, Meredith Gartin, Meskerem Glegziabher, Joseph Hackman, Ashley Hagaman, SeungYong Han, Kim Hill, Katie Hinde, Daniel Hruschka, Megan Jehn, Erika Jerme, Kelly Knudson, Liza Kurtz, Jonathan Maupin, Charlayne Mitchell, Monet Niesluchowski, Christopher Roberts, Alissa Ruth, Roseanne Schuster, Rachel Scott, Rhian Stotts, Cindi SturtzSreetharan, Sarah Trainer, Ben Trumble, Polly Wiessner, Deborah Williams, and Abby York.

Over the years many other colleagues have provided thoughts, feedback, and conversations that helped shape the idea and then the form of this book, including Richard Aguilar, John S. Allen, Ernesto López Almada, Gro Amdam, Eileen Anderson-Fye, Meg Bruening,

Elizabeth Capaldi, Deborah Carr, Monica Casper, Neetu Choudhary, Matt Gervais, Jennifer Glick, Ellen Granberg, Lance Gravlee, Craig Hadley, Jessica Hardin, Jennifer Hooks, Bonnie Kaiser, Dong-Sik Kim, Brandon Kohrt, Tom Leatherman, Linda Lederman, Shir Lerman, James Levine, Arulraj Louis, Brenda Major, Chris McCarty, Stephanie McClure, Amy McLennan, Randy Nesse, Steven Neuberg, Peggy Ochandarena, Ivy Pike, Danielle Raves, Eric Robinson, Asher Rosinger, Lori Roust, Fernanda Scagliusi, Larry Schell, Karen Schmidt, Roger Sullivan, Angelina Sutin, Seline Szkupinski-Quiroga, Nicole Taylor, Janet Tomiyama, Wilda Valencia, Lesley Jo Weaver, Andrea Wiley, and Heather Worth. We are extremely grateful to all for sharing their expertise and thoughtful criticism. We are also very thankful to science writer Laura Sessions, director of The Write Stuff, for her careful and important work in editing the overall text, Alyssa Lindsey for editorial support in preparation of the final submission, and our editor Robin Coleman.

In the obesity research discussed in the book, we particularly benefited from the financial support of the Virginia G. Piper Charitable Trust and the ASU Office of the Provost for the Mayo Clinic–ASU Obesity Solutions initiative. Alex's conceptual work for chapter 6 was supported by a visiting fellowship at the Center for Advanced Studies in Oslo. In the water research we discuss, we benefited from funding provided by the US National Science Foundation (BCS-0314395, BCS-1759972, DEB-1637590, SES-1462086).

Our initial collaboration, focused on rethinking how anthropologists do cross-cultural research, was seeded in 2008 by a special five-year award to "Late Lessons in Early History" for the President's Strategic Initiative Fund at ASU through the support of ASU's president Dr. Michael M. Crow, a powerful driver of the types of transdisciplinary scholarship this book engages. Much of our more recent scholarly work discussed herein occurred in the context of two research collaborations that we have together led over the last decade: Mayo Clinic–ASU Obesity Solutions (on weight) and the Global Ethnohydrology Study (on water and hygiene). Undergraduate students, hailing from a diversity of places across the globe, have worked as research lab apprentices helping with the important tasks of data management and checking on both those projects; other students helped crucially with summer data collection across the years in places around the globe. Many were part of the global health undergraduate program at ASU. This book was written with those amazing, energetic, determined students in mind. Their drive to create a just and effective world through better ways of addressing health and healthcare gives us great hope for what lies ahead.

LAZY, CRAZY, AND DISGUSTING

Why We Wrote This Book

What This Book Is About

Emma had never smoked.[1] When she was diagnosed with metastatic lung cancer at age 52, she was both angry and confused. She knew women her age who had been diagnosed with breast cancer. They had outpourings of warmth and support from families, friends, and strangers, and embarked on healing journeys full of Facebook likes, flowers, and home-cooked casseroles. They were hero warriors, applauded for their bravery and strength. She had entered a different and darker cancer world, one festooned with shame and blame instead of survivor ribbons. As she put it: "If it's not pink, there's just not a lot of sympathy out there for you." She knew others suspected she must have done something wrong, like sneaking cigarettes. After all, innocent people don't get lung cancer. For a while, Emma made sure to tell everyone "I have cancer, but I never smoked." But it didn't seem to help. Finally, she began to simply say she had cancer in her bones. Then came kindness, compassion, and encouragement.

Emma's struggle to be seen as worthy of care, to have her illness understood by others as the unfair burden she believed it to be, was created by one of the greatest successes of modern public health: the campaign against tobacco. In the first half of the twentieth century, new methods for manufacturing tobacco, the invention of the safety

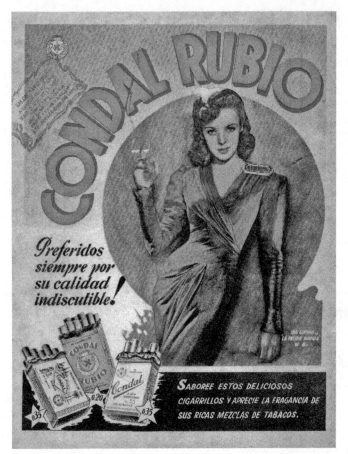

Figure I.1. Latin American tobacco advertisement, 1936. From the collection of Stanford Research into the Impact of Tobacco Advertising

match, and mass media advertising created a new market for smoking (figure I.1). It sold the idea of cigarettes as affordable, accessible, and pleasurable. Movie stars lit up seductively. World leaders puffed as they signed historic deals. Doctors extolled relaxation benefits, lit cigarette in hand. Smoking became the cool, social, modern, sexy, grown-up thing to do. By midcentury, the majority of Americans, Australians, and Europeans were smokers.

But in the second half of the twentieth century, the health consequences of tobacco became clear. The discovery that it causes debilitating lung disease and painful deaths from cancer prompted energetic, sustained public health efforts to push people to quit. Smoking was banned from public places. Tobacco advertising on television and in magazines became heavily controlled. Smoking products were highly taxed. But quitting a nicotine addiction is really, really hard.

So, public health pulled out the big guns and used *stigma* to turn public attitudes. By stigma, we mean the process by which people become classified within society as less valuable, undesirable, or unwanted.[2] Public health messages changed tobacco from fragrant to foul.[3] But it wasn't just the smoke that was demonized. The smoker, too, became newly defined as disgusting and unwanted. They became *stigmatized*, marked as weak and selfish and otherwise morally valueless by their habit. They were recast in the public imagination as villains who were committing the slow murder of those around them with their toxic, secondhand smoke (figure I.2).

Smokers found themselves the targets of intense judgment and rejection from many around them. People looked at them sideways, refused to kiss them, and instructed them to step outside. In the face of this new and powerful stigma, many smokers found the means to quit—no matter how physically difficult. By the turn of the millennium, public health declared the campaign against tobacco a success. The power of stigma had changed entrenched behaviors, overcome addiction, and saved millions of lives.

But this is where the success story of smoking starts to turn sour. And it is where our book—about the complex, dangerous dance between stigma and public health—begins. Fervent anti-smoking attitudes can harm Emma and others like her. In a world where disgust toward smokers is expected and normal, people find themselves blamed for having illnesses associated with smoking (even if they had never smoked). They endure particularly deep guilt and shame if they actually smoked and anger at the implication if they didn't. They are treated as exiles among the healthy.[4] Compared to people struggling with thirteen other common forms of cancer, not surprisingly those with lung cancer have the highest level of depression during and following treatment.[5]

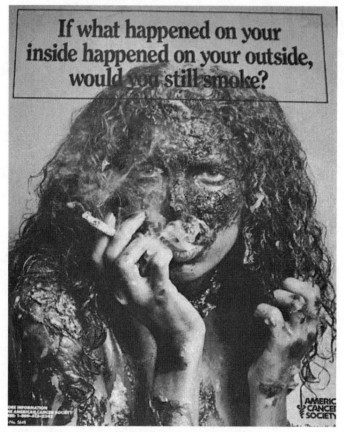

Figure I.2. American Cancer Society anti-smoking advertisement. From the collection of Stanford Research into the Impact of Tobacco Advertising

Dodging the dreadful judgment, many don't tell their friends and family about their illness or avoid medical treatment altogether. They die sooner than they should. Their deaths come with less love, support, and caring than they deserve, or would otherwise get, if their diagnosis was for a less stigmatized disease.

And, not everyone stopped smoking. The new stigma was especially effective in helping people higher on the socioeconomic ladder to give up tobacco. Those with more money, contacts, and education had more practical means to help them quit. They could get smoking cessation drugs from their doctors or attend classes paid for by their employers. In contrast, smoking rates remain as high as ever in the lowest-income sectors of the wealthy nations. These more vulnerable citizens are now the primary target of a powerful tobacco industry desperate for customers. In lower-income communities in the United States, for example, tobacco billboards are larger and much more plentiful, there are more stores selling tobacco, more point-of-sale promotions touting discounts on price, and greater social pressure to smoke.[6] The act of smoking itself also provides a way to cope with the stressors of being at the bottom of the social and economic ladder. It helps to stave hunger, soothe stress, and make people feel connected to others sharing their problems.

At the same time, smokers in these communities have morphed into the primary target of extremely aggressive, shaming anti-smoking public health campaigns. In breeding the self-perception that smokers are useless and ignorant, self-efficacy—the sense we can do anything to change—is undermined. So, instead of helping the lowest-income smokers to quit, the anti-smoking campaigns may solidify the very behaviors they are trying to discourage. As yet, public health has absolutely no plan for how to solve this wrinkle in the anti-smoking success story. And the lack of effort to fix it reminds us that in public policy, some lives (and deaths) matter more than others. The lives of "stupid" smokers are viewed as less worthy of public attention and investment than those of "blameless" middle-class women with breast cancer.

Why We Wrote This Book

Smoking offers a powerful parable of how using stigma as a public health tool to change social norms can go terribly wrong for those who are already at the margins of society. Understanding how and why this happens has been a major motive of our program of research over the last decade. But it wasn't tobacco that first spurred our quest to unravel and expose the ways that stigma and global health can derail each other. It was a simple news item that crossed our desks in 2007, covering a, at the time, new approach to improving sanitation in rural villages in Asia. It was called Community-Led Total Sanitation (CLTS). CLTS provided a very low-cost solution to the challenge of getting people to build and use toilets. The intervention was designed to trigger disgust toward those who defecate outdoors or don't wash their hands, thereby nudging social norms to make people want to be more sanitary. The goal was certainly noble, since diarrheal disease is a major childhood killer and better hygiene saves lives. And early studies of CLTS showed fabulous results: People who were shamed were frantic to build toilets, regardless of the effort or cost needed.

What stunned us about CLTS was the explicit use of shame as a tool in a public health intervention in such clearly vulnerable communities. These interventions were being rolled out in the types of places we have worked as anthropologists throughout our entire careers: impoverished communities with no running water and no sanitation infrastructure. Having lived with people living in poverty, we knew that they battled constantly to be respected as dignified and valued members of society. And we knew too well what the negative consequences of shaming interventions could be. In our fifty combined years of fieldwork studying the human dimensions of health struggles, we had so often seen how shame was emotionally devastating. In our work on family planning in small Micronesian villages in the remote central Pacific, we had heard the stories of women desperate for children, shaking as they explained their failure as wives and daughters because of their inability to get pregnant. In our studies of water insecurity in dusty South American informal settlements, we had listened to fathers, their heads dipped with humiliation, as they told us they felt ashamed because they couldn't bring home enough money to buy water for their families. Observing in schools in the United States, our hearts went out when we saw children being cruelly bullied by classmates because of their body size. Shame dramatically undermines human dignity, our very sense of our basic worth in the world.

But shame itself—while dreadful and painful—is not what concerned us most about CLTS. It's what happens when you mix it with poverty or any other marginalized social status (like being old, female, gay, transgender, HIV positive, or an undocumented immigrant, to name but a few). Then shame quickly and easily cascades into stigma. As this book makes clear, it is stigma that is truly health damaging and deadly. And so, we were acutely aware of the possible risks inherent in CLTS just because it had the potential to create and amplify stigma. We asked each other, incredulously: Didn't these global health campaigners see how easily these new interventions could go awry? Hadn't they thought that they might end up heaping more stigma on the poor? Weren't they afraid that the marginalized, the powerless, those without the capacity to push back would be most damaged in their wake? And how could they embrace these risks when they didn't have solid evidence that the intervention itself made people healthier over the long term? Had nobody warned them that stigma born of shame can be a global driver of illness? It seemed the answer was "no." And so, reading about that one case of CLTS training in Bangladesh opened a whole new focus area for our work together.[7]

The CLTS approach, using disgust and shame to encourage healthy handwashing in poor, rural villages, has a thoroughly explicable, sensible, and sound scientific basis, rooted in the massive success of those anti-tobacco campaigns. Once we started digging, we found so many other examples of how using stigma as a tool to push health behavior change had backfired. Like the early days of the HIV/AIDS epidemic in the 1980s, when there were calls for forced quarantines to protect the "good" people from the "bad" ones. At that time, blame for the disease was placed squarely on those living in ways deemed dangerous and morally wrong: drug users, men having sex with men, and sex workers. This stigma against people most at risk of HIV helped fuel the epidemic. Understanding the dreadful social damage that being diagnosed would inflict, people acted sensibly: They avoided HIV testing.[8] Millions of lives were lost as a result.

And the story repeats, over and over again, with different diseases and different vulnerable groups. It's all right there in front of us, but mostly invisible because no one is looking for it. Recent campaigns to promote child health across the globe, for example, provide a very

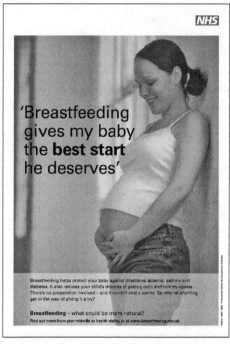 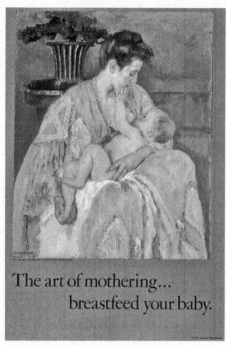

Figure I.3. While encouraging healthy behaviors, "breast is best" health messages can also inadvertently suggest to women who formula feed that they are failing as mothers and possibly hurting their babies. *Left*, National Health Service, UK; *right*, US National Library of Medicine

particular image of a "good mother" as someone who breastfeeds (figure I.3). By promoting this as a social expectation, mothers who formula feed their children can feel anxious, guilty, angry, uncertain, and ashamed. These feelings of stigma mean those unable to breastfeed because of health issues or rigid work conditions don't seek or get the information they need on safe formula feeding—and their babies are more likely to get sick as a result.[9]

But a larger issue remains, even as sanitation scholars are starting to document the harmful stigmatizing effects of CLTS, and child and maternal health advocates are beginning to push back against some of the "breast is best" messaging.[10] Identifying the problem *after* the interventions are over is simply too late. The damage is already done. And our ability to fix things after the fact is especially stymied when working in communities already made vulnerable by poverty, disease, or political marginalization to begin with. So, at one level, our book presents a basic, necessary message for anyone working in health: Watch out for stigma. It's a basic, fundamentally unrecognized driver of what happens in health.[11] Yet many health practitioners barely even recognize it, even within their own work. In the field of global health, where many of the most important efforts are happening in the poorest communities, the implications of this blind spot easily escalate.

Many of those who choose healthcare as a profession care deeply about the people and communities they serve. And because stigma especially attaches to disease, health professionals are in a unique position to see, challenge, and redress it. Those who work in global health are often particularly and intimately aware of the challenging conditions in which many people must struggle to live each day. Doing business as usual, believing—at the very least—they are doing no harm, can mask damage being done. We wrote this book to help make stigma more visible. The hope is much of that unintended damage can then be better anticipated, planned for, and so avoided. People who work in the health fields are always in prime stigma territory for one basic reason: Disease is a particular magnet for stigma exactly because stigma tends to attach to "what matters most" to people.[12] Illness—the suffering that disease brings[13]—is a fundamental part of the human condition that we are all afraid off and desperately want to avoid. It speaks to our deepest fears and anxieties—of pain, helplessness, and death. Thus, all healers and caregivers, who work intimately with people who are sick, are situated at the front lines of stigma.

But this book isn't intended just as a conversation with people who manage disease or disability every day, whether in Toronto or Timbuktu. We humans are a universally, inescapably judgmental species. Our readiness to stigmatize is part of that. And so, it invades all our lives, all the time. We struggle daily to avoid the many possible labels that we believe will make others reject, avoid, and otherwise discount us: "crazy" (mental illness in our family), "slutty" (histories with herpes or abortion or multiple sex partners), "lazy" (weight), "hopeless" (disabilities), "weak" (smoking), "out of control" (drinking), "unmanly" (impotence), or "unfeminine" (infertility) to name just a few. Discerning how stigma works and what to do about it is relevant to everyone who cares what others think, wants to belong and be valued, and seeks to treat others fairly; in other words, it's relevant to all of us.

Medical anthropology as a field has produced outstanding ethnographic work that is relevant to our understanding of health-related stigma.[14] Some excellent case studies are provided in Paul Farmer's analysis of how structural stigma creates additional vulnerabilities around HIV/AIDS in Haiti, Cassandra White's analysis of leprosy in Brazil, Marcia Inhorn's work on women's experiences with infertility in Egypt, Charles Brigg's exposition of how stigma shaped a cholera epidemic in Venezuela, João Biehl's detailed study of living with disability in Brazil, Sarah Trainer's study of patients with very high body weight in an American hospital, and Joan Ablon's action-focused work on impairment disability in the United States.[15] Each can be an enriching single case to be read as a companion to our more synthetic treatment herein. Erving Goffman's earliest work on people with mental illnesses confined to asylums, which later came to utterly define the construct of stigma for many social scientists, is also recommended reading.[16]

Yet, even if they have produced some really detailed, sophisticated individual case studies of the damage done by stigma in the last several decades, and most is focused in some fashion on disease and disability, anthropologists have engaged surprisingly little in general theory building around how stigma and health collide.[17] While sociologists and psychologists have long embraced that stigma is a key defining concept in their fields, anthropologists have not. Even so, our conclusions in this book of the broader damage that stigma does in the contexts of global health will likely be no surprise to anthropologists, particularly the idea of stigma as a profound form of human suffering. The most basic but broader question of *why* humans stigmatize is one our field should have much to say about. This is because the stigma is a complex cultural phenomenon, tightly tied into our social norms—our shared ideas about how things *should* be. Public health provides a particularly rich context to advance this needed agenda, if only because—as noted—almost all our stigmas are rooted in some fashion in our fears of contagion and disease. The comparative, integrative approach we take in this book, placing the ethnographic cases into a wider picture, is designed to fill this gaping hole.

In the social sciences, there is still significant conceptual confusion about what stigma is, what it does, and—especially—what we should do about it. On one hand, political economic analysis shows how the "stigma power" of disease can be harnessed institutionally to control and exploit people and communities. Stigma can be used as a tool to block access to quality healthcare and the basic resources like food and water that are needed to support health. This creates deadly cycles of illness that reinforce the existing institutions and power structures. In this view, properly formulated global health efforts are *solutions* to the problem of stigma—the means to break the cycle of poverty and illness and allow people to thrive. On the other hand, evolutionary-minded scholars highlight the connection between the human tendency to create social and physical distance from things deemed as disgusting, improper, or undesirable. This approach highlights the need for adaptive strategies to avoid contagion in our hypersocial species. In this view, *stigma is the solution* to the problem of global health. This more biological orientation also helps explain why stigma exists even when there seems to be nothing ostensibly gained, no "stigma power."

Between these two views lies the unchartered territory that must be navigated to create truly just, sustainable health. And this is the terrain where this book is purposefully situated. By integrating and balancing these two, quite different, perspectives—in the context of what we observe on the ground as anthropologists who work in the global north and south—the goal is to dig deeper and create a new and globally oriented synthesis to understand stigma in the contexts of global public health. We are reaching toward an understanding of the intimate, pervasive, powerful—and significantly more complicated and often unrecognized—relationship between stigma and health.

How to Navigate the Book

The book is designed to build an argument: that global health processes often unwittingly create and reinforce stigma, and this undermines global health's basic goals to create both health and justice. An important point in navigating the text is that our goal is to integrate and explain what we have learned from our five combined decades of experiences on the ground with communities across the globe as field-based medical anthropologists.[18] Our ongoing conversations (and writing) with social scientists and public health colleagues, and our long-term familiarity with the scholarly literature, deeply informs our perspective.

The book is, as such, not intended to be a systematic review of all the available literature, although certainly it is fully informed by it. We use ethnographic cases to illustrate key points, either from our own research or that of other scholars. Ethnographic research involves many methods, but the most important is participant observation: Researchers live in the research site and experience firsthand the problems they study. Ethnographic research produces rich descriptions of social and cultural phenomena, often as part of a mixed-method study design. Many ethnographers supplement their participant observations using surveys with selected samples of respondents, social network analysis, experiments, direct observations, and even biological data. When ethnographic exemplars (cases, stories, examples) are presented, they have undergone an extensive process of qualitative analysis. In this way, they are not merely anecdotes; rather, they are selected based on their representativeness of the results of rigorous fieldwork. Also note, while the people whose stories we highlight in this book are all real, the names we use are not. It is standard practice in ethnography to use pseudonyms.

The arguments we make are also informed fully by current evidence from epidemiology and other quantitative (empirical, numerical) research in social science. Qualitative and quantitative approaches are complementary and, broadly speaking, excel in advancing different kinds of research. Qualitative approaches are excellent for exploratory research, particularly focused on new or poorly studied social phenomena, cultures, meanings, and lived experiences. Quantitative approaches are ideal for testing hypotheses around well-understood social phenomena and for producing findings that generalize to a population. Each basic approach to data collection and analysis can yield different—often complementary—results even when conducted in the same place on the same topic.[19]

Our own field research typically combines the two. We were lucky to be trained in both, and we recognize the analytic advantages of having different forms of evidence to draw on simultaneously as we draw our conclusions. For example, we often do larger-scale surveys or systematic behavioral observation (quantitative), alongside in-depth interviews (qualitative), assuming we will find our slightly different things from each and working through the implications of that as we interpret findings. However, most other current research relevant to stigma in global health is based on one tradition or another, and part of our process of building the arguments herein were to make informed, integrative decisions in the space between them.

To this end, from the perspective of the reader, we settled on an approach for presenting evidence in this book that gives primacy to ethnographic cases. The epidemiological or other quantitative data that supports or balances is, by contrast, more often presented in the endnotes. This isn't to say the numbers aren't crucial to the argument being made. This was done to make it easier (and more enjoyable) for readers to follow what is a complicated set of ideas. But for those used to weighing epidemiological or other numerical evidence, constant reference to the notes will likely be important to a satisfactory and convincing read.

There's another purposeful reason we give primacy in the main text to the case studies and then provide the parallel numerical evidence as the support, rather than the other way around. It's actually much easier to use numerical evidence and scientific language to discuss global health outcomes. But there is plenty of evidence that tells us humans learn better and understand more deeply when information is transmitted through storytelling. Sharing the evidence in this way, we believe, is the best way to help readers understand in a more nuanced way how stigma harms lives. And that shared understanding is absolutely crucial to spurring a wider desire and willingness for the necessary social change.

We also don't want to overextend pathos. To get people to care about stigma and suffering (and to fight for or donate to related causes), scholars, nongovernmental organizations, and journalists sometimes deploy a trope called "development pornography" or "poverty pornography."[20] This is the use of evocative language or images to sensationalize people's struggles and shame, such as photographs of starving children. It's meant to shock readers—who may otherwise ignore social problems every day—into caring. But as social scientists who are driven by a desire for proper and balanced evidence, we work hard to be truthful about painful realities without, at the same time, sensationalizing in ways that sacrifice people's right to dignity. This sets a very high bar to clear when writing about stigmatized conditions and behaviors, but we've done our best to meet it in setting a balance across both different forms of evidence and different ways to communicate around suffering as we present our case. We will let you, the reader, be the judge of how well we have succeeded.

The core three sections of book are where the argument is detailed. Each addresses a different major and current public health challenge as a way to focus the case studies. These parts are identified, in the titles, by some of the moral judgments that they evoke: community sanitation ("disgusting"), obesity ("lazy"), and mental illness ("crazy"). We chose health challenges that we know are ridden with stigma and already locked-in with poverty globally. They were also selected because they are the topics we have grappled with at various points in our own research histories. These illnesses are chronic, complex, and lack simple cures: Exactly the sorts of global health challenges that are the greatest magnets to the powerful and damaging social suffering that stigma creates. Each part can be read alone as a case study on stigma related to a specific global health challenge but, read sequentially, they provide the explanatory basis for why we are firm in our conclusion: Avoid using stigma as a tool to influence health behavior changes.

In part I, "Disgusting," we use the case of sanitation efforts in international development to explore and explain how and why humans so readily stigmatize, how this derails ongoing public health efforts, and why this process invariably runs downhill to particularly damage the most vulnerable people in society. We open chapter 1 with a deep dive into the campaign that first shocked us into our current focus on stigma a decade ago: CLTS efforts to rid the world of open defecation. Global sanitation and hygiene efforts are a cornerstone of global public health.

The case of sanitation also helps us understand why dignity matters greatly to a good life and good health. Dignity is about feeling that you bring worth to the world and that worth is recognized by those around you. Stigma is so painful because it replaces dignity with rejection, causing people to feel shame, self-blame, and doubt. It tells us we contribute nothing of value and our struggles are meaningless. It is one thing to be hungry or thirsty or dirty, but it is another to be told your suffering is your own fault. To have a sick child is emotionally devastating, but to know that others believe that sickness implies your failure as a parent moves the dial on that misery up several notches. In chapter 2, we use evidence from our own recent cross-cultural field research on community hygiene norms to expand a key point: Our fearful reactions to visible disease markers are easily projected onto people as stigma. We show that—crucially—this projection of stigma onto others is more about our desire for prestige, and much less about our innate fears of disease. In chapter 3, we move from the cultural to the structural, identifying how stigmatizing ideas about dirt and contagion become embedded in public health responses to epidemics: conflating dirty things with dirty people. Examining two diseases often associated with lack of hygiene and poverty—cholera and leprosy—we show how stigma within global health practice piles more and more shame, illness, misery, and suffering on the least powerful.[21] The ability to ignite self-doubt and shame makes stigma an amazingly effective tool for pushing people down, out, and away from others. Applied to whole groups, we show how stigma can be used as a chillingly effective political tool. More, because structural stigmas make people feel hopeless and reinforce the status quo, these stigmas make activism or other forms of fighting back difficult.

In part II, "Lazy," we explore how *new* stigmas enter global health, and outline why that happens so easily, using the case of anti-fat views embedded in efforts to combat obesity and related chronic diseases. This shows how completely *new and powerful stigmas* can emerge because of our medical and public health efforts, ultimately undermining their most basic goals: to reduce disease and erase health disparities. In chapter 4, we outline how anti-fat attitudes are deepening and spreading globally, creeping into the public imagination and our daily lives almost invisibly but very powerfully. Obesity is a great example to understand that the human propensity to stigmatize is often implicit and unquestioned; stigmatizing others often feels morally right, and we assume is obviously true. It is just what we do, so we have a hard time recognizing it as anything other than business as normal. We also then, in chapter 5, explain how efforts to address obesity globally are probably driving new epidemics of disordered eating and depression. This is because public health approaches to obesity prevention are seeded with stigmatizing notions of individual responsibility and blame, despite growing scientific evidence that the basis and solutions of obesity lie in structural factors—like how our work, schools, and neighborhoods are organized. Chapter 6 then applies this recognition to anticipating some of the downstream effects of the national-level anti-obesity campaigns that are being rolled out globally, including how they might very well lock in stigma and poverty. The invisibility of stigma to global health practitioners is, we argue, a major part of the problem.

In part III, "Crazy," we examine mental illness to consider why destigmatization is so very difficult. The stigma of mental illness has long been recognized by mental health professionals as a major impediment to its treatment. Yet despite decades of hard work, the goal of destigmatizating mental illness has proven elusive. In chapter 7, we explore some of the more common approaches to destigmatization that have been applied, and why most are sadly doomed to fail when dealing with chronic, complex illness. In chapter 8, we challenge a myth that permeates the stigma literature: that small-scale societies are exceptional places where mental illness stigma is less of a problem. We reexamine the ethnographic evidence and we argue that this leads to two damaging views: that mental illness in small-scale societies isn't as bad as elsewhere and that changing cultural ideas about mental illness is a relatively simple fix.

In chapter 9, using the case of depression, we continue to build our argument for another wrinkle to addressing stigma—how stigmas tend to beget other stigmas. Stigma doesn't just sicken us by blocking access to health services and discouraging us from seeking help. It does much more. It makes us more vulnerable to poverty and its effects, destroying our health through diet, overwork, indebtedness, and stress. It adds additional emphasis to one of our key messages: that stigma, once attached to conditions and groups of people—and most especially to those living in poverty and otherwise marginalized—is incredibly hard to shift. It can trigger anxiety, depression, and other mental illnesses that can lead to waves of suicide. The case of mental illness also paves the way to consider, in the conclusion, some new ways of thinking, with more optimism, about possible ways forward. We find that there are important lessons to be drawn from this research that *can* help us build global health programs that are less stigmatizing.

The final chapter, our conclusion, focuses on what can be done to prevent, challenge, and fix stigma. We focus on really difficult cases: sanitation, mental illness, obesity—the chronic, widespread health challenges that we highlight in the book. These problems can seem intractable, maybe even hopeless. But we believe there is good reason for overall optimism. There are cases where we have seen real reduction in stigma making a significant impact on both the experience and the course of disease, especially specific infectious diseases that have a cure, or at least a reasonably good prognosis. We discussed the case of breast cancer above, a good example of how shifts in popular culture have reduced fear, changed the way breast cancer patients are viewed and treated, and thus transformed how the illness is experienced. Activists, doctors, and public health workers have purposefully and successfully removed much of the stigma around HIV/AIDS, through large-scale, targeted, public education campaigns about the transmission of the disease.[22] This has led to more government and private investments in basic research and clinical trials, thereby making drugs more affordable and accessible to those who need them.

In considering how to navigate this book, we want to pause on an important point. Having worked on these problems for a long time, we know that they can be, in turn, depressing and disheartening. It's important to acknowledge that, for people living with stigma (or even just researching it), it can be hard to overcome feelings of despair. This is something we talk openly about with our students and colleagues. And there are lots of things we do, big and small, to help us maintain our energy and passion for working on this issue. One important thing for us is community—having people around who share our dedication to health and justice. We get really angry sometimes, and we try to be open about that, too. Making jokes helps. Another is staying healthy—we both struggle with this one, but we try to remind each other to take a break, exercise, go to the doctor when we're sick, and just take care of ourselves. We've found that therapy, meditation, and other forms of mental healthcare are especially important for people who live with stigma day in and day out. Last, and this is probably the hardest one, we have to remind ourselves to embrace hope. It's always there—change is happening all the time—but sometimes we forget to look.

Change can, and often does, come from stigma sufferers themselves. Working as anthropologists, over the decades we have observed, up close, how people come together to push back against—and rise above—the most seemingly overwhelming obstacles. In our work on obesity, we have marveled at committed fat activists harnessing social media to challenge the status quo of how people living with obesity are portrayed in media and on television. In Bolivia, we have seen impoverished communities pull together and rise up against powerful government and multinational companies to return control of water to the people. Similarly, in Kiribati, we have watched the citizens of a small and powerless country learn how to push back to demand global redress for climate change, as their low-lying villages flood with rising tides and their fresh water supplies dwindle. We never underestimate the power of activists and encourage global health professionals to partner with these brave stigma fighters.

Looking more broadly at modern history, we know truly profound societal stigma transformation is possible. Before 1973, homosexuality was classified as a psychiatric disease and being openly gay, even in the most liberal social settings, would likely cost you your job and your family. In many states, men having sex with men were at risk of criminal prosecution and imprisonment. But by the end of the first decade of the new millennium, half of all Americans had advanced on supporting symbolic and legal changes (such as the right to marry) that underpin a growing view that sexual orientation should not be a basis for moving people down and out of society. That shift—from society viewing same-sex love as wrong and stigmatized toward embracing same-sex partnerships as belonging and inspirational—to us, is an incredibly hopeful message of what is possible.

Stigma is, most simply, a process of being labeled as socially unwanted and what flows from that. But, as you will discover through the pages in this book, it often manifests as a complex, tricky, wicked problem[23] that defies simple descriptions, single theories, or straightforward fixes. So, at the very end of the book, in an appendix, you can find a general primer to help navigate this complexity. It is there as a reference for those who want to understand more about how we think about stigma, such how it tends to work, make sense of confusing terminologies, and outline some of the core scholarly theories applied to it. It is mostly intended to help as a general reference on stigma when the book is used as a text, such as in anthropology or global health classes. You don't need this primer to be able to understand the book.

Skimming it at the outset and then referring to it as you proceed will help you better navigate the book. Reading it at the end will deepen appreciation for the theory woven through the text, providing a better theoretical lens with which to understand the arguments we make and the cases we highlight.

Part I

Disgusting

1

Dealing with Defecation

Global health work is sometimes truly disgusting. To save lives, you have to deal with shit—literally. In northern Mozambique in 2016, we visited Pemba, a small, beautiful, rambling, friendly East African port town, prone to both droughts and floods. Stretched along the world's third-largest bay, wooden and metal huts crowded amid thick-trunked, bulbous baobab trees and skinny, tall coconut palms. As we went house-to-house interviewing, we kept our eyes carefully focused on every step. Feces were everywhere. Mozambique has, as a result of concerted public health efforts, seen a shift from 40 to around 70 percent of people reporting they use toilets in recent decades. But in areas like Pemba, outdoor, or open, defecation (OD) also remains normal, acceptable, and common (figure 1.1).[1] Of the households surveyed at the time of our visit, 80 percent had some form of toilet in the home as a choice, but the others had only their yards, the river bank, or the mangroves at the water's edge. For those who did have access to a toilet, another 11 percent admitted they never use it at all, preferring the open-air options.[2] One-third of all the people we interviewed didn't agree that enforcing toilet use would increase the health of the community, and they were three times more likely to be those who practiced outdoor defecation. Alex discovered all this in the most personal way when—exiting a taxi—she accidentally fell into a street culvert used for the purpose.

From a public health perspective, exposure to human waste is a terrible, dreadful disease disaster. Just one tiny gram of feces contains up to ten million viruses, ten million bacteria, and millions of parasitic eggs.[3] In the low-lying, coastal neighborhoods of Pemba, the arrival of monsoon rain marks the time of greatest risk. Flooding dislodges feces. Carried in water supplies, cholera-infected drinking water causes severe dehydration, while typhoid causes body-racking fevers. Untreated, both can kill quickly and painfully. Waste from OD means flies carry diarrheal disease into homes and onto people's food. Seeping into soil, the eggs of nutrient-sucking, cognitive-impairing hookworms hatch and chew their way into our bodies through bare feet.

These less deadly infectious agents inhibit the gut's capacity to absorb nutrients. They cause diarrheas and other sickness that undermine a person's capacity to do work or get an education. In children, they even cause stunting and damage normal cognitive development. In fact, something like 5 percent of all deaths globally are caused by what is termed "unimproved sanitation,"[4] and mostly young children in low-income countries in Asia and Africa are affected.[5] These are the deaths that would be preventable through basic sanitation measures that hygienically separate people from their waste, such as with a flushing or composting toilet and an adequate handwashing station.[6]

So, if there are so many good reasons to practice basic sanitation by building and then using a toilet, why isn't everyone in Pemba on board with making building and using toilets a priority? First, building latrines requires supplies that cost money that many families don't have. Second, water is often far away or expensive to buy. Getting enough water to flush and to clean can make maintaining toilets a real burden. Public latrines may help solve this in some places but are often unsafe for women to visit on their own after dark, putting them at risk of assault.[7] And there are other explicable, cultural reasons in Pemba that—even if people do have access to toilets—they nonetheless choose to defecate in the open. In our interviews, people explained the pleasure of the ritual of daily walks to the beachfront. It is a chance to unwind and catch up with friends. Sitting all alone in a

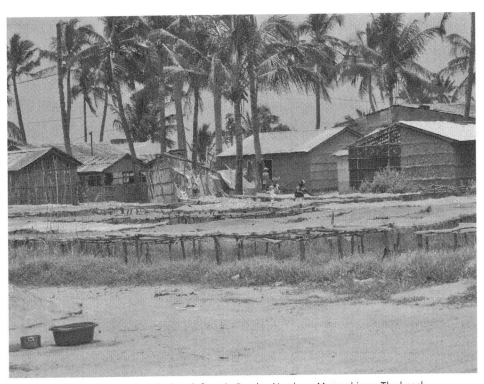

Figure 1.1. Houses line the beach front in Pemba, Northern Mozambique. The beach is used as an open defecation site. Photo by A. Brewis

smelly latrine can't do that. To people in Pemba, someone who defecates at the beach or in the tidal mangrove swamp is being social and practical, not gross and disgusting.

Similarly, in Butaritari in Micronesia—a low-lying Pacific atoll where Alex lived in a rural village for a year in the 1990s—there is a long history of open defecation. There, too, people wandered to the shoreline to defecate. Squatting with backside out to sea—even waving as people go by—was seen by the villagers as hygienic, relaxing, and appropriate. But, obviously also at odds with public health goals to prevent the diseases caused by open defecation. And so, at the time Alex was living there, foreign aid workers arrived, erecting a proud concrete toilet block right in the middle of the main village to deal with the problem. Residents were given instructions on the need to clean the stalls daily and held an opening ceremony complete with ribbon-cutting. But right after the experts left, the island council president locked the doors. He explained, "How else will we stop people from dirtying them?" People were blasé about using them anyway. One woman mused, as she wandered back down to the beach to do her business, "Why would you want all your shit piled in one place? That's disgusting." Another pointed out the unnecessary work of hauling water to flush, explaining "Why bother when you can use the beach, and the tide will come in and wash the shit away for you? It's better that way, anyway."[8]

As anthropologists well know, these refusals to use toilets or to wash hands are not simply ignorant objections. These reflect core values about how people understand what is clean and proper, our *hygiene norms*. Norms are shared, learned, cultural understandings of what behavior is permitted and what is not. These hygiene norms are often informal and unwritten, things we learned as children. Consider the cultural rules about the right way to clear excess snot from the nose. In France, sniffing it back in is preferable, but this is disgusting to many Americans. In the United States, blowing it into a tissue is considered polite, but entirely gross to the Japanese, who translate *hanakuso* (handkerchiefs) as "nose waste." But in all three societies the rules about what you should do with snot support the idea that rather than letting it drip profusely from your nose and onto others, it should be discretely removed. Mostly, it's a good thing that all societies have hygiene norms, because they are a key social mechanism to keep us separated from the body fluids and other things that might carry disease.

Our shared hygiene norms may guide and even compel our public behavior. Handwashing by using soap, rubbing the hands, and washing with water reduces the risk of spreading fecal disease by up to half. Currently, 19 percent of people in the world reportedly wash their hands after using a bathroom. The higher rates in higher-income countries, like Australia, the United States, and the United Kingdom, clocking in around 50 percent, reflect prevailing hygiene norms that say "it's disgusting not to wash your hands after toileting." Yet, that still means as many as half of those in places with ready access to soap and water, who know this social rule and understand the health benefits, actually don't always wash their hands at home.[9] Even doctors in the best healthcare systems don't always wash their hands between patients as recommended. In one study, UK healthcare workers were told that they were being directly observed, but there was no mention that the study was about handwashing. They found doctors washed their hands less than half as often as would be medically indicated (nurses and other allied workers did much better at 75 percent).[10]

But, when others are watching, like when using a shared public bathroom, people seem more likely to hand wash, because they are concerned others will think them unclean. The change is modest perhaps but still significant: One recent experiment in Argentina placed a complicit user in men's campus restrooms and then compared users' behaviors to those left alone. The presence of a peer increased handwashing rates from 66 to 79 percent.[11] Leveraging our quest for social desirability (and conversely avoidance of social shame) to help change our bathroom behavior has emerged recently as a central tool in global sanitation efforts.

The Practical Uses of Disgust and Shame

Like other governments everywhere facing persistent open defecation, Mozambique and Kiribati both recognize that improving sanitation is crucial to their national development efforts.[12] Until a decade or so ago, most sanitation projects in lower-income countries focused on physically building toilets and washstands and supplying soap. This was often combined with top-down poster or radio advertising campaigns about the health benefits of using them.[13] Sometimes the projects worked, sometimes they didn't. But, overall, these concrete solutions helped save millions of lives. However, something like 60 percent of people globally still live without a flushing toilet, and just under a billion people globally are without any type of sanitary toilet facility at all and defecate outdoors. Public health still has much work to do to reach the United Nations sustainable development goal of 100 percent access to adequate sanitation by 2030. The main snag?

It is inordinately expensive to build a toilet and washstand, or even just to provide soap, for those two billion more people. Someone has to pay. And there's a second snag: Sometimes you build the toilets but then people choose not to use them.

A little over a decade ago, global health experts realized that perhaps *changing* community *hygiene norms* could be the key to solving both problems, and thus the global challenge of open defecation. First designed by livestock specialist Kamal Kar in Bangladesh, Community-Led Total Sanitation (CLTS) emerged as an effort to activate communities to *want* to build and maintain their *own* toilets. It is an approach designed specifically to nudge local hygiene norms to make open defecation and failures to handwash socially unacceptable. Pragmatically, it is a much cheaper approach for advancing public health, because the costs and effort of building toilets and handwash stations are passed on to communities themselves.[14]

How does this work? As CLTS literature explains it, you "leverage the crucial role that social pressure and social expectations can play in sustaining new sanitation behaviors." Put more simply: You teach that it is *disgusting and shameful* if you don't use a toilet or don't wash your hands.[15] CLTS begins with community meetings that focus on

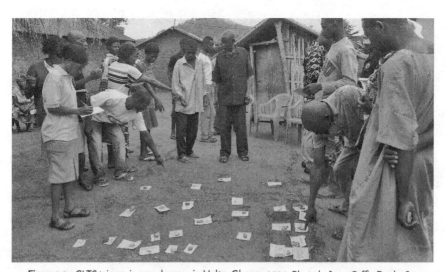

Figure 1.2. CLTS triggering underway in Volta, Ghana, 2014. Photo by Jesse Coffie Danku Sr

"triggering" exercises (figure 1.2). These are designed to elicit disgust toward the behaviors of open defecation by connecting it directly to instinctive aversions to body waste. Like in the Chibwe village in Mozambique, where the residents drew giant maps in the sand and each identified, with piles of gray ash, their own defecation sites. Then they together calculated that their ninety-three homes would produce 84,723 piles of feces per year.[16] CLTS isn't just about individual behavioral change; it is about creating a powerful emotional shock that will change community norms to make unsanitary behaviors (like open defecation) socially unacceptable. The value messages conveyed in CLTS programs are that people who wash their hands are better, more deserving, and have good reason to be proud. This has a mirrored effect on those who don't (or can't) meet the new standards, reinforcing the idea that they are, by implication, less deserving, less valuable, and less necessary to the community. CLTS is social engineering, designed to redefine who is designated as "clean and good" and who is "disgusting and bad" (figures 1.3, 1.4, & 1.5).

The explicit point of all this is to create new forms of collective moral outrage, so villagers will rally to humiliate any resident who doesn't then build and use a toilet. That is, they build new forms of shame. Two years after it was introduced in 2008, some 1.2 million people had been "triggered" in Mozambique,[17] and 466 villages were declared open defecation free (ODF).

These shaming strategies even lead to communities inventing new forms of severe hygiene self-policing. In Sierra Leone, for example, CLTS has led to communities adopting fine systems. Being caught defecating in the bushes, not having a handwashing facility at home, failing to report a broken latrine to the local sanitation committee, or not showing up for monthly community toilet-cleaning duty can lead to US$1 fines.[18] This is no small amount of money in Sierra Leone, where the per capita GDP is less than $500 a year.

Buoyed by such visible proposed successes, even more extreme shaming tactics are now being designed and deployed, like the Super-Amma soap handwashing campaigns in India and Africa.[19] As with CLTS, SuperAmma provides no toilets, no water, nor even soap.

Instead, the hallmark is the public pledging ceremony, in which women commit to handwashing as the right thing to do and receive a certificate as a reward. The names of the pledgers are displayed publicly along with photos of public figures washing their hands. Non-pledgers become shamed by their absence.

A recent review of best practices for promoting handwashing concluded that interventions based on disgust were among the most effective ways to promote public health, at least over the short term.[20] It is less clear if the behavior change triggered by these disgust- and shame-based campaigns is sustained over the long term, or if they are directly linked to their capacity to reduce disease exposure. Scientifically, the evidence seems equivocal at best.[21] Evaluations of the SuperAmma campaigns concluded, "[W]e are not able to distinguish the effects of the different components of the intervention, for example, whether disgust, nurture, status, or affiliation was the most impor-

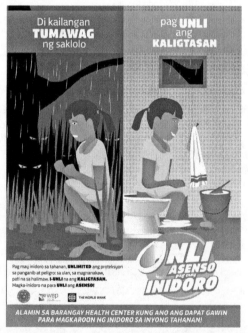

Figure 1.3. Sanitation poster from the Philippines, leveraging the fear that open defecation puts children at risk of malevolent spirits, dangerous people, and wild animals. Used by permission of the Water & Sanitation Program, World Bank Group

tant driver of behavior change. Neither can we say for how long the effects of the campaign will last."[22]

Regardless, this cheap and relatively easy approach to sanitation is spreading. Governments in low-income countries also remain enthusiastic about CLTS and similar approaches because shaming people into building and paying for their own toilets is so much cheaper than providing them with the required hardware. In the last several years, CLTS and similar programs have been rapidly scaled up, growing into one of the most widely used approaches for improving sanitation in the lower-income countries of the world. They are now applied in some seventy countries, mostly in Africa and Asia, including new and rapid expansion into South America.[23]

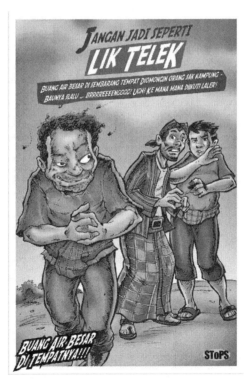

Figure 1.4. This poster from Indonesia translates as "Defecating in the open makes you the talk of the whole village. The stench is . . . Yuck! Ugh! Flies follow everywhere you go!" Used by permission of the Water & Sanitation Program, World Bank Group

Why It Works

There are good reasons that disgust and shame can be powerful tools in the sanitation arsenal. Both are strongly felt, evolved human emotions. Along with fear, anger, sadness, and happiness, they are observed across all human societies.[24] Whether in Papua New Guinea or Palm Springs, people display the same physical reaction of disgust to things that gross them out. Mouths gape, lips curl back, noses wrinkle, breathing speeds up, hearts beat faster, stomachs sour, and nausea rises. We recoil from food wriggling with maggots, the sight of oozing pus, and the smell of vomit. Even imagining disgusting things can make us distance ourselves from what might be dangerous. Close your eyes and imagine a cockroach swimming across a bowl of chicken soup. Then think of picking up a spoon and beginning to eat it.

Disgust is potent because it's designed by evolution to elicit the instinctive reactions that keep us alive.[25] Humans are omnivores that will eat a stunning array of different species; we are not like hummingbirds born knowing exactly what we should eat. Rather, our brains are geared to try many foods. But we have to be careful what we put into our mouths in particular, as it is the easiest way for pathogens or poisons to enter our bodies. Disgust at things that smell or look wrong (like a cockroach swimming in our soup) helps balance our sensation-seeking tendencies to try out new foods against the risk of eating things that make us sick or kill us. This explains why the facial expression of disgust is the same as what happens when we taste foods that are too bitter. It also accounts for why our strong disgust reactions appear around ages 3–4, right when young humans begin to seek out and eat food by themselves.[26]

Humans are particularly revolted by body excreta like pus and feces, the very materials that most often carry infection. For much of human history, there was no knowledge of pathogens nor medical preventions like vaccines. An instinctual wariness of people who had overt signs of disease, like vomiting, diarrhea, or dripping sores, might have been a lifesaving. Having a gut reaction—one that makes us want to avoid the types of people that disgust us—can help us make fast decisions about what might be dangerous and thereby keep us safer.[27] Disgust, reinforced by local hygiene norms, tells us what and who to avoid, keeping us healthy—a "behavioral immune system" if you will.

Consider the lives of many women living with obstetric fistulas. These fistulas result from abnormally extended birth labor.[28] The baby's head stays pushed against the mother's pelvic bone and prevents blood flow for so long that her soft tissues begin to die. This can create a leaking hole between the rectum and the vagina. Fistulas are uncomfortable, messy, and identifiable by their smell. Because an obstetric fistula usually happens in the rural reaches of the poorest countries, where medical care is far away, only a small percentage of women get the relatively easy surgically fix. The rest (something like two million women globally) must struggle with chronic incontinence for the rest of their lives.[29]

The smell and mess of leaking feces are hard for others not to recoil from; this makes sense since other people's feces can easily transmit disease and so humans are well-served to instinctively want to avoid handling it. But that social rejection by others is socially distancing and shaming for affected women. Once loved and valued, women with fistulas find those around them withdrawing. They are often forced to eat, pray, and sleep alone. Their husbands even divorce them. One 36-year-old Eritrean woman explained, after living with a fistula for fourteen years, "You cannot even get close to someone to be comforted."[30] This shows the very tight and mostly unconscious connections between instinctive disgust, social rejection, and feelings of shame that coalesce around our hygiene norms, or how we define what clean smells, looks, and acts like.

Shame here, like disgust, is an intense and powerful emotion. But it engages our failures to meet social norms rather than physical revolt. It activates when we are told or believe that we are failing to live up to ideals or the expectations of others. It causes us to hide our faces, contract our bodies, and is often followed by an uncomfortable, rising hot sensation and tears. In small doses, feelings of shame remind us to attend to social expectations and to modify our actions accordingly and work to fit in. It helps smooth the challenges of being a social species that requires cultural rules and a high level of cooperation to survive. For actions like using a toilet or washing our hands, it can be a useful push for prompting and reinforcing sanitary behaviors that keep us physically safe. But when you are fundamentally unable to meet those basic norms of smelling acceptably clean—such as when you have an untreated fistula—it can be devastating, even life destroying.

This is because when shame and disgust collide, humans too easily connect instinctive feelings of revulsion to *moral* ideas about people's worth.[31] It allows, permits, and even encourages cruel mistreatment. It releases people from an obligation to show empathy. For example, all societies have some taboos around the handling of menstrual blood. But the idea that reproductive-aged women are polluting of all those around them for several days of the month is learned.[32] In western Nepal, menstruating girls are accordingly banned from school to keep the other students safe.[33] Their prospects for a better life are dashed as their education is undermined.[34] Women of all ages are made to sleep in sheds so they don't contaminate others living in the house. They are denied adequate bedding; the reasoning is that bedding contaminated by menstrual blood is polluted and can't be used by others. Nutritious milk, yogurt, butter, and meat are withheld from menstruating women, for fear they will contaminate it or the animals it came from. And this can kill. Like it did for newly married Dambara Upadhyay who died cold and alone in a hut behind her in-laws' house, cast out only because she was menstruating.[35]

In large doses, when disgust transforms into rejection, shame, and enacted stigma, it can do serious and systematic damage. Importantly, too, judgments attached to public or known transgressions of hygiene norms get applied differently on the basis of social distinctions, like gender, but also income, age, or ethnicity. Immigrants sweat and stink from a day of "dirty" manual labor, while the elite glow healthfully after an afternoon of vigorous, "clean" exercise at their expensive gym.[36] Disgust and shame might be evolved, but the depth and meanings of the feelings they evoke are clearly shaped by, not just local cultural values, but *who* within society is being shamed. And this is exactly where the real problems of CLTS lie.

The Problems with Disgust and Shame: Or, Why CLTS Needs to Stop

In the Micronesian village of Butaritari where those earlier toilet-building failures happened, Community-Led Total Sanitation was introduced in 2013.[37] There, CLTS implementers also led "walks of shame," pointing out the excrement on the ground as people followed them on a tour of their village defecation spots. They collected human feces during the walk, later placing them in a water bottle and offering it to people to drink. Thoroughly disgusted and embarrassed at the idea they were "eating their own shit," families rushed to build new pit latrines.

But that rush can derail if the latrine building experts are left out of the loop. This happens easily with CLTS, since the point is to avoid the cost of not just materials but technical expertise. A couple of years after CLTS was implemented in Butaritari, a visiting United Nations sanitation specialist discovered the new cesspit toilets were polluting the precious, scarce fresh water lens under the atoll,[38] the main water source on these dry, low-lying islands. Once again, people eschewed the toilets. However, the new shame they had learned through CLTS toward open defecation meant they now didn't want to be seen by others defecating on the beach. Instead, they hid in the bushes. The tide used to carry the waste out to sea twice a day, as it had done for thousands of years. Now it is piling up on land instead, more likely to transmit hookworm from person to person or infect the fresh water supply with the giardia or dysentery amoebas that cause diarrhea.

This suggests that the shame generated by CLTS may endure even if the behavior change doesn't. Some CLTS funders have hinted that the shame that it generates might not always be a desirable outcome, because it can generate these types of publicly acceptable exclusions of people that don't—or can't—follow the newly instigated hygiene norms. One evaluation of CLTS programs noted that that "messages

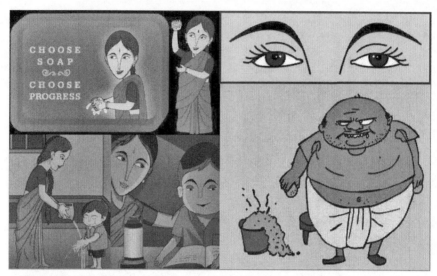

Figure 1.5. Materials from a Community-Led Total Sanitation campaign in rural India. Reproduced from A. Biran, W. P. Schmidt, K. S. Varadharajan, D. Rajaraman, R. Kumar, K. Greenland, et al., "Effect of a Behaviour-Change Intervention on Handwashing with Soap in India (SuperAmma): A Cluster-Randomised Trial," *The Lancet Global Health* 2 (2014): e145–e154

have been seen as too blunt and have had to be modified to create triggers which do not excessively shame and disgust." A 2014 UNICEF report suggested that these approaches could cause those unable or unwilling to meet new community norms to "become excluded (banished or subject to penalties) from their community where the rules around latrine construction and open defecation are strictly enforced."[39] They noted, though, that they hadn't actually observed any cases of banishment, so maybe the problem wasn't too serious.

As anthropologists, we think this misses the point entirely. These types of hygiene stigmas rarely lead to total physical banishment like that endured by some menstruating women in Western Nepal. Rather, they more often trigger lower grade, but still humiliating, forms of social exclusion like being mocked, ignored, or otherwise mistreated— even done with the "best" of intentions. This is exactly what happened in the case of Subornokhuli, Bangladesh, a tiny farming and fishing village of rice paddies, orchards, and bamboo groves. CLTS arrived in the community in full force, with the goal to ensure every home had access to a proper toilet. Local sanitation committees, led by the more outgoing and often wealthier women, became the organizers and created a mobile court. They withheld old-age pensions or seized work carts to demand the payment of fines. It was even announced that girls raped while defecating outside would no longer have the support of the local legal system.

The poorer families were paid to act as "social engineers" to do the triggering work. They went through the village with loud speakers to announce new penalties for open defecation. The village children got so riled up that they jumped out of bed early every morning to catch people defecating in the bushes. They blew their CLTS-provided whistles to alert others to offenders. They threw stones at people squatting in public. They mounted small flags on any feces they found, labeling them with the names of the offenders. Responding to the widespread and public shaming, people tried to put up new latrines as best they could.

But what about those who couldn't afford to build toilets, such as the poorest of the poor? Determined to make their community open defecation free, the committee of village elites took it upon themselves to install cheap, flimsy latrines made of local bamboo in the offending households. And then they handed the recalcitrant households the bill to pay. Within just a few months, CLTS was declared a roaring success. Every household now had access to a toilet. The village committee swelled with pride at their clean, open-defecation-free village.

In 2008, monitoring and evaluation specialist Amina Mahbub arrived in Subornokhuli to study what had happened in the intervening six years.[40] She was especially interested in how the most vulnerable households had fared in the wake of CLTS. She found the poorest families had installed latrines they just couldn't afford. Their motivation was fear of monetary and social punishment. Most concerning was the new humiliation of their daughters. They were being cruelly teased at school for being dirty and disgusting. The poorest families in Subornokhuli, the ones who were essentially destitute to begin with, now found themselves utterly stigmatized. They had no choice but to find a way—any way—to pay for that toilet. Some families even went without food as a way to meet the debts incurred by the forced build. Others were forced to take out loans with extremely high, predatory interest rates.

Several years later, with no money to repair them, many of the toilets were no longer functioning. The bamboo had rotted away. The formerly zealous children had grown bored of chasing excrement and moved on to new excitements. Many had reverted to open defecation. CLTS had created other problems, too. Those who didn't have extra land to place the toilet had erected it on a public pathway or on someone else's land. This had created new, bitter conflicts between neighbors. Despite all the effort, the village's sanitation "success" hadn't lasted,[41] but the debt, conflict, and new sanitation stigma left in its wake did.

This brings us to the most important point about the potential of Community-Led Total Sanitation to cause harm. Although CLTS seems to be one way that global health practitioners can deliver improvements in toilet facilities, it does not deliver its improvements in ways that benefit everyone equally. From such examples as Subornokhuli, it is easy to see how CLTS can too easily undermine people's basic dignity and punish the poor for their own misery. Those most likely to be damaged by shame-based social engineering are those who are poorest and otherwise marginalized to begin with, like women or minorities. Those most affected are already without a voice, at the bottom of the social ladder, unseen by those who oversee the interventions.[42] This may also explain why CLTS interventions have been found to be most successful in places where working toilets are already widely available and just a few community members still need to be encouraged to use them (almost always the poorest families). It is easier for the masses and those with more power to shame the few with less.

Proponents of CLTS argue that if it is implemented *exactly* as designed, it won't cause these types of humiliation. Instead, it can empower the poorest by building pride and the realization of self-potential.[43] The problem, though, is that "communities" have all sorts of divisions across spectrums of wealth, political power, gender, and religion. Our colleague Kathleen O'Reilly, a geographer who has worked in India on sanitation for almost twenty years, is an expert in understanding how social inequalities shape people's ability to get and use toilets in India. In one study in West Bengal, O'Reilly selected groups of villages that recently won their state's Clean Village Award. The community leaders had used their own versions of CLTS "shock and shame" methods to stop open defecation, such as photographing and threatening people. O'Reilly documented how these campaigns disproportionately targeted the poorest households. However, she also found it wasn't just those living in poverty that were harmed by CLTS methods. All sorts of social divisions—including language, caste, indigeneity, rurality, and widowhood—were being amplified and reinforced by the shaming interventions.[44]

CLTS may only work exactly as intended if whole communities— especially people with higher incomes, social class, and social status— take collective responsibility for supporting and assisting the poorest and most marginalized. For example, resources could be pooled to build and maintain shared latrines for all. Unfortunately, forming these types of collective action institutions isn't usually part of the design of these programs.[45] Not everyone is able (or even wants) to work together, especially on a new challenge that is not based in a rich history of local values and traditions.

Most concerning, CLTS programs have not been monitoring these damaging impacts much, if at all.[46] Moreover, it is not even clear, stigma aside, that the overall strategy is actually working especially well as a sanitation intervention. In a recent review that assessed the amassed scholarly studies claiming successes—evaluating each on the criteria of quality of reporting, effort to minimize bias, and appropriateness of the conclusions drawn for each—it seemed that the current evidence base was in fact extremely weak.[47]

At the same time, helping those with the greatest need to build toilets isn't enough on its own either, given the deep social meanings people everywhere place on body waste. Some form of influential, safe health education is needed as well. India has persistent OD, despite decades of energetic sanitation interventions that includes affordable options for pit latrines. A recent synthesis of multiple lines of evidence for rural India (including national surveys, local surveys, and long-term ethnographic fieldwork) concluded the problem remains that manual latrine cleaning is seen as the work of *dalits* (untouchables). For all those in higher castes, clearing your own waste from a toilet is thus extremely degrading. Even if you have the money to pay for the toilet itself, it costs a lot to have a *dalit* come from the city to empty it. And having the latrine in the house, proximate to the places people eat, is also ritually polluting. OD is thus perceived as "cleaner."[48]

There are other, potentially non-stigmatizing, ways to educate around sanitation, that could similarly trigger positive change because they leverage different innate human propensities. One that we find especially hopeful is efforts that engage our curiosity and love of play. In an internally displaced person (IDP) camp in Iraq in 2018, a team of public health experts and social scientists piloted a handwashing intervention that embedded toy animals within bars of soap. Through the transfer of glitter when high-fiving, targeted school-age children were taught how handwashing removed transmissible germs. Compared to those who got only plain soap and a standard—less fun— sanitation training, the children who experienced the toy-glitter intervention were four times more likely to be washing their hands with soap a month later.[49]

The Big Questions

Global health is about advancing health as a human right. So, CLTS raises some difficult questions about balancing the need for equality and dignity against health itself. Even if CLTS was 100 percent effective at getting every person in the world a workable toilet, is its social damage justifiable? Is sanitation for all worth the painful, damaging humiliation and rejection of some?[50] This is a difficult moral and philosophical question. As anthropologists, who deal in the downhill effects of damaging stigma, we argue that programs like CLTS that engage disgust *and* shame should be completely abandoned—at the very least until the social stigma and longer-term sanitation impacts of CLTS and similar programs are adequately tracked and addressed. Sanitation experts driven to save children's lives from infectious diarrheas by any available means might conclude differently.

But all this begs a more fundamental question: Why is this happening at all? Why does disgust jump from being applied to objects (feces) to staining people's social identities to the point they are discarded as worthless? Why are hygiene norm violations, like defecating in the wrong place or menstruating at all, such a focus for this? And, why do ruinous processes always seem to flow down social hierarchies, piling up on the least powerful? It's a story rarely told in public health, but it needs to be. The answers can be gleaned from anthropological studies conducted in communities across the globe and are the focus of the next two chapters.

The Bottom Line

There is no doubt that ensuring adequate sanitation saves millions of lives. Reducing open defecation and increasing handwashing are rightly a pragmatic, central goal of global health action. But sanitation projects that leverage our innate disgust reactions can have a dark side for global health efforts, inadvertently proliferating shame and rejection. The damage accrues particularly to those already socially or economically disadvantaged. We suggest avoiding shame-based approaches entirely in sanitation behavior-change efforts and, instead, innovating strategies that draw on our very best human tendencies. These are likely to be much less destructive and may even work as well or better to promote sanitary health.

2

Dirty Things, Disgusting People

British anthropologist Mary Douglas returned from research with the Lele in the Belgium Congo, taking time out from fieldwork to raise three children (figure 2.1). The most influential work of her career, *Purity and Danger* (1966), was a study of ethnographic and historical literature on dirt, hygiene, and contagion written while full-time parenting. It clarified that in all societies people are fundamentally concerned with what and who is dirty ("polluted") and what and who is clean ("pure"). Essentially, as she put it, "dirt is matter out of place." Taboos are the social rules that tell us the things that we must absolutely avoid, because they are the most contaminating and dangerous of all. The notion that hygiene norms, including taboos (prohibitions) about what to eat, how to bathe, or who to avoid, are essentially prescriptions for health is counter to Douglas's basic thinking. To her, hygiene norms and the practices they shape are mostly idiosyncratic; that is, what is and what is not defined and acted on as dirty is all relative.

She certainly agreed the health advantages were absolutely conferred by some religious rituals, like regular bathing mentioned in the Old Testament. But, as she bluntly put it, Moses was no "enlightened public health administrator."[1] Historical hygiene norms like the monthly seclusion of menstruating women in hamlets in New Guinea, growing ultra-long fingernails in ancient China, and emptying

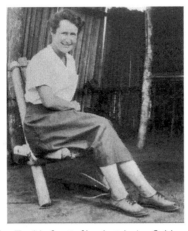

Figure 2.1. Mary Douglas (Tew) in front of her hut during fieldwork with the Lele, Zaire, circa 1950. Photo by W. B. Fagg, © RAI

chamber pots out windows onto the street in medieval Europe might be healthy, or they might not be. If hygiene norms have a purpose, Douglas reasoned, it is to create and reinforce the broader social order. They shore up the subjugated public roles of women, or the power of the elite. If such norms also happen to confer any health advantages, this just enhanced their symbolic (social) power.

What's the Danger?

Stigma itself was not a concept that Douglas addressed head-on in *Purity and Danger*. She danced around it, though, and we can learn much from taking a whirl with her. India's Havik Brahmin belief system was one of the historical cases Douglas analyzed. Nearly all social interactions were organized into three designations of ritual purity, Douglas argued. The highest ritual status was "pure" and is appropriate for worship. The middle "neutral" state was good for interacting with others but unfit for worship. The lowest state was "impure" and unfit for interaction with others. The boundaries between these pure and polluted states were policed by a range of core disgust concerns involving food, bodily fluids, physical contact, and bathing. To maintain a pure status, you had to bathe three times a day, as well as after touching blood, pus, animal waste, leather, your own saliva, or anything touched by someone in an impure state. The lowest untouchable status could contaminate a home, a meal, a rope, and straw flooring by just touching them. The state of being unclean (and unable to become clean) proves a dominant social identity. As a result, for Douglas, hygiene norms and their violations took a central role in creating social stigma and in policing social status in a hierarchical society—with no clear and apparent link to health at all.

When we started our own ethnographic work focused on stigma a decade ago, we were eager to learn what field-based research other scholars had done testing Douglas's ideas in the fifty years since *Purity and Danger* was published against the evolutionary predictions about hygiene norms as a "behavioral immune system" discussed in the prior chapter. We were surprised by the answer: not much. There has been an open debate about the degree to which cultural notions of disgust and stigma are linked cross-culturally to disease risk or other health advantages, but no clear empirical demonstration.[2] If Douglas was right, there should not be a very tight link observable between hygiene stigma and infectious disease risk. Stigmatization would be about maintaining social boundaries, not disease prevention. If the evolutionary theorists are right that hygiene norms are all about disease, we should expect to observe cross-culturally a clear link between hygiene stigma and infectious disease risk. In this case, stigmatization would be about disease prevention, not about managing social power structures. Lots of people had ventured guesses and constructed arguments based on interesting examples, but there wasn't much empirical evidence to guide our thinking on stigma either way.

So, frustrated by a lack of research to draw on to answer our questions, we did what any self-respecting anthropologists would do. We headed off to do fieldwork. We went back to three global sites where we have worked previously. Americans have been described by anthropologists as a society unusually culturally obsessed with the need to smell good, have clean teeth, and other markers of extreme levels of hygiene, so the US case was an important one to include as well, and we did that work just up the street from our offices in Arizona.[3]

What We Did

For the last decade, we have had enormous fun, and learned a lot, together running a large, cross-cultural, field research project we call the Global Ethnohydrology Study.[4] The research is a transdisciplinary team effort to study cultural norms about water. We work at highly varied sites across the globe, with each site carefully selected to advance our understanding of the role of water scarcity, economic wealth, and other political and ecological factors in shaping cultural norms.[5] Our goal is to develop basic theories and practical insights about how people cope when water is scarce.

We tackle a different global health or environmental challenge each year, such as understanding cultural views of the basic causes of waterborne disease or people's worries about future climate changes.[6] In 2015, with the assistance of some fifty Arizona State University global health undergraduate students, we set off to collect data on hygiene norms and stigma from four hundred people living in culturally distinct sites in four corners of the world (figure 2.2). At each research site, we began by asking people about their daily hygiene habits, such as when and how often they washed their hands and showered. We checked if they had soap, water, and handwashing facilities. We collected people's responses on the "disgust" scales that evolutionary scholars had developed by showing them twenty different photographs of insects, diseased bodies, and contaminated objects.[7]

We also asked people about a long list of possible hygiene norms, and how they felt about others who didn't follow them. We asked about things such as their reaction to someone who rarely cleans their bathroom at home, wears the same clothes two days in a row, or does not wash their hands after using the toilet. Douglas considered how hygiene norms related to what people perceived as *dangerous*, not just dirty. To capture this, we asked people how much distance they needed from people they knew were behaving in less sanitary ways, such as not washing their hands after going to the bathroom, not washing their clothes regularly, and so on.

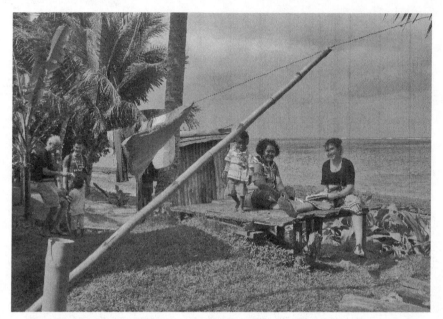

Figure 2.2. Conducting interviews to elicit hygiene norms in Fiji, 2015. Photo by D. Williams

Then we asked people to describe in detail what someone who was unacceptably dirty would be like. People talked about things like goopy eyes, greasy hair, foul clothing, and dirty nails. Then we asked them *who* this person was. That is, we wanted to know if they viewed this person as just being physically dirty or labeled them as part of stigmatized groups and (if so) what those groups might be.

Where We Went

We selected four global sites for our hygiene stigma research: Fiji, Guatemala, New Zealand, and the United States. These locations were picked to provide a range of risks posed by sanitation-related illness from high to low.[8] If sanitation mattered, we reasoned, we would see more stigma and cultural concerns around hygiene norm violations in the sites with greater sanitation-related disease risks.

In Guatemala, where sanitation-related disease rates are the highest of all four sites, we did research in a small, rural town called Acatenango in the center of the country. Our collaborator Jonathan Maupin has been doing participant observation on healthcare in the same village for over a decade. He has known the place well since childhood, as his grandfather founded the clinic there.[9] In Acatenango, people get their water from wells. Waterborne parasites like amoebiasis are very common and cause diarrheal disease, vomiting, and malnutrition. To be safe, water must be fully treated.

In Fiji, we did interviews in a small, tight-knit village that sits on the edge of the Pacific Ocean. We have been visiting the same village each summer for some fifteen years with our global health students, planting mangroves and helping with reef rebuilding to address climate change threats. Alex first visited the village some thirty-five years ago, when she was herself an undergraduate. In the interim, the village has developed their own community water system by damming upriver. Most houses have easy access to taps that bring the water into the village. Some houses also have their own rainwater tanks. Even so, water availability can be intermittent and water quality is spotty. In years of flooding, typhoid becomes a concern. Milder diarrheal disease from fecal contamination is also common, likely due to inadequate handwashing. Alex brought her daughter on one visit and spent days nursing her through dreadful, bright green, rotovirus-induced diarrhea. On another trip, a large set of our students staunchly endured a nasty wave of cramping, vomiting, and diarrhea thanks to what turned out to be a dose of campylobacter.

In the United States, we conducted research in Phoenix, Arizona, where we both currently live. Phoenix is a sprawling desert city, where searing hot concrete is decorated by blowing dust. While municipal water authorities manage water wisely, the threat of water shortages and drought is ever-present. The extreme dry heat means that we all carry bottled water with us in the summer. At the end of a long day, we come home and find our clothes baked in dried sweat. In the summer, our feet crack and chap after exposure to the dry heat.

We regularly experience the symptoms of dehydration, such as headaches and confusion.

In New Zealand, Alex's home country and the site with the least infectious disease risk, we interviewed people in the capital city of Wellington. In reputedly "clean and green" New Zealand, the municipal water supply is almost always safe and most people drink directly from the tap.[10] New Zealand has some of the highest handwashing rates of any country; the hygiene norms are well-enforced. Illness and death related to water, sanitation, and hygiene issues are some of the lowest in the world.

Comparing the scores on reported hygiene and disgust measures across the four sites, we found a lot of consistencies, despite all these differences in basic sanitation and infectious disease risk (table 2.1). One unexpected finding across sites was that consistent handwashing after toileting was reported to be significantly lower in the US site (Phoenix, Arizona) compared to the other three sites.[11] However, taking a summary score of frequency of basic hygiene behaviors (an array of handwashing, bathing, house cleaning practices), average levels proved much the same in all four sites.[12] New Zealand respondents had slightly lower disgust sensitivities compared to the other sites, meaning they found pictures of the gross items less off-putting. Those at the Guatemalan site felt more susceptible to infectious disease, which makes sense given that rates are higher in Guatemala. Guatemalans also identified a preference for a greater social distance from people who are "dirty" than the other sites.

In analyzing the data of what people said when asked to describe hygiene violators, we focused our analysis particularly on gender differences between what people say about men versus women. Why? Globally, women (and mothers in particular) are more likely than men to be responsible for water procurement—and to be blamed and shamed when homes or children fail to meet cultural standards of cleanliness, washing, or water use.[13] Beyond this, much greater hygiene expectations are placed on women than men in most societies. Women are expected to invest more time and money in extensive grooming activities of hair, skin, nails, and smell.[14] Therefore, if dis-

TABLE 2.1.
Summary measures of hygiene behaviors, disgust sensitivity, preferred social distance, and perceived disease vulnerability across the four study sites

	Viti Levu, Fiji (N = 59)	Acatenango, Guatemala (N = 65)	Wellington, New Zealand (N = 82)	Phoenix, United States (N = 61)
After using the toilet, how often do you wash your hands?				
"Always"	93.3%	96.9%	89.2%	68.9%
Hygiene Behavior Scores: Based on average site response across twenty-six different household and personal hygiene behaviors from 1 ("never do it") to 4 ("always do it").				
Men	3.27 (.34)	3.4 (.31)	3.01 (.37)	3.12 (.29)
Women	3.44 (.27)*	3.53 (.23)	3.07 (.34)	3.12 (.44)
Disgust Sensitivity Scores: Based on average site reaction to nine photos of potentially disgusting objects, from 1 ("not at all disgusted") to 5 ("extremely disgusted").**				
Men	31.8 (11.4)	30.6 (14.3)	19.4 (11.3)	22.3 (7.8)
Women	35.5 (13.1)	34.6 (13.7)	25.9 (11.5)*	31.7 (16.3)*
Perceived Vulnerability to Disease Scores: Based on average site reactions to 15 items asking about germ/contagion fears and avoidance (possible range 0 to 90), with higher scores reflecting higher perceived susceptibility.**				
Men	44.8 (16.2)	43.7 (13.4)	37.1 (8.3)	40.4 (4.7)
Women	47.6 (13.4)	48.4 (16.2)	39.1 (9.0)	40.9 (1.4)
Social Distance Scores: Where lower average scores represent increased preference for greater social distance from someone who is unclean.				
Men	2.31 (.65)	1.73 (.66)	2.27 (.75)	2.22 (.69)
Women	2.15 (.69)	1.80 (.79)	2.25 (.75)	2.06 (.82)

*Statistically significant gender difference based on t-test.
**Statistically significant difference across sites based on one-way analysis of variance (ANOVA).

cernable cross-cultural patterns in disgust, hygiene norms, and stigma exist, we reasoned, they would probably manifest *most intensely* in the data from and about women.[15]

What We Found
What Do Hygiene Norm Violations Look Like in Each Country?

Imagine a woman that is unclean in a socially unacceptable way. What does she look like? What is it about her that makes her unclean? Imagine her hair, her face (eyes, ears, nose), her mouth, her skin, her hands, feet, underarms, and clothing. How can you tell that these parts of her body are unclean? This is exactly what we asked women to talk to us about at the four research sites. Keep your own answer in mind as we compare how other women answered these questions around the globe. While there were some differences in the kinds of clothes and grooming expected in each country, the answers were fairly uniform in identifying socially unacceptable hygiene norm violations.[16] The violations tended to be related to body odor, visible dirt, and yellowed teeth.

In Guatemala, where deaths from lack of sanitation are most common, we interviewed María Fernanda, a 43-year-old married woman.[17] An evangelical Christian, María Fernanda worked as a cleaning lady and characterized herself as lower middle class. Her home had a television as a luxury, but no cell phone, internet, or other technological facilities. Her family often lacked water and sometimes couldn't afford to eat the foods they preferred. She didn't care much if people didn't bathe daily and was not worried about being around other people who didn't wash their hands. María Fernanda's description of a woman who was unclean in a socially unacceptable way was typical of those we collected in Acatenango. She described a woman with a dusty, filthy face; disheveled hair; and unclean skin. Her hands, María Fernanda told us, would be sooty, dusty, and dirty. Her mouth and her armpits would smell bad. Her undergarments would be filthy and sweaty.

In Fiji, we interviewed Esiteri. Her responses were typical for women from her village. A 33-year-old, she characterized herself as a married, middle-class, stay-at-home mom. Her village home was described as comfortable, with a TV, internet, and a cell phone. She always had enough food, but, like others in the village, she sometimes struggled to get enough water from the community water tap. Nevertheless, she reported, she kept a well-maintained home with a clean bathroom. She emphasized that she washed her hands meticulously and was careful to be clean when she was preparing meals. She was clear that she wouldn't want to be around people who didn't do the same. In her description of someone who is unclean in a socially unacceptable way, she listed red eyes, a drippy nose, dirty ears, and yellow and missing teeth. "This woman has big and scary hair," Esiteri said. "She has dirty, hairy armpits. She has scabies on her skin. She has long fingernails and long toenails."

In Phoenix, we talked with a 22-year-old teacher named Brittany. She identified as white, university-educated, and upper class. Brittany had a well-equipped house with every amenity, abundant food, and plenty of heated water. She admitted she was relatively lax about hygiene norms, only occasionally washing fruits before eating and utensils after handling raw food. She said she sometimes reused clothes and underclothes, and sometimes skipped showers. She said she felt comfortable having people who had violated a range of hygiene norms in her personal space. Brittany described a woman who is unclean in a socially unacceptable way as having bad dental hygiene and strong body odor. This woman, Brittany said, would have nails that are long and unkempt and feet that are dirty and smelly. She would have a dirty face that was breaking out with acne and smudged with dirt. Her hair would be a knotty mess and her clothing would be dirty and ripped.[18]

In Wellington, we talked with Vicky, a 27-year-old hostel assistant. Vicky was unmarried, university-educated, and came from what she described as an upper middle-class family. She lived in a comfortable house with every modern amenity expected in a high-income country like New Zealand, with plenty of food and hot running water whenever she needed it. Vicky was not overly fussy about handwashing and was okay about being around other people who didn't wash their hands either. Vicky's description of a woman who is unclean in a socially unacceptable way described sun-marked, brownish skin and dry lips, unshaven underarms and bare feet. She imagined gray, messy hair that was dirty and knotted and nails that were long and kind of beaten. She said that the woman would not be fully dressed.

When we compare across the sites, we get different stories about where the blame lies for the violation of hygiene norms. In Guatemala, the woman was ascribed less personal blame because poverty was the compelling reason. In Fiji, the blame mostly fell to the family,

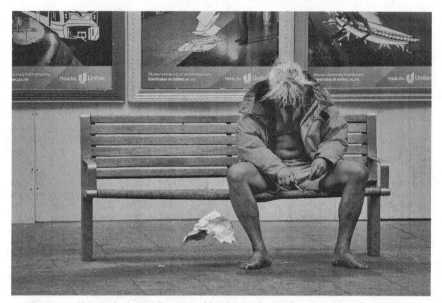

Figure 2.3. This stock photo taken in Auckland, New Zealand, in 2017, identifies the subject as "homeless man eating on the street." Intended for use by media outlets, the composition of the photo was unlikely to be consciously stigmatizing. Yet it reinforces the connection of homelessness to both poor hygiene and social rejection. © Shutterstock

who should have cared better for the woman. In the United States, the person was to blame but was excused in part by bad luck and misfortunate. Finally, in New Zealand, the most stigmatizing blame was placed on the person themselves, with fewer mitigating excuses. Looking at the full dataset, too, we find that blame for hygiene violations varies across the sites but is lowest in Guatemala and highest in New Zealand.

Yes, but Are These Hygiene Norm Violations Stigmatized?

The next question we wanted to answer was whether these hygiene norm violations were merely seen as a distasteful and transitory state of affairs or if they were stigmatized. Put another way, are hygiene norm violations linked to devalued social identities? To answer this, we asked our respondents to tell us the backstory of the socially unacceptable, unclean woman they had imagined.

In Guatemala, María Fernanda didn't think there was much she needed to say beyond "peasant." She described the unclean woman as someone who was poor and worked harvesting coffee in the country-side. Alternatively, she said, she could also be someone who is lazy, careless, or lives on the street.

In Fiji, Esiteri told us a story of an old woman with no relatives who love her. She was pushed out of society with no one to depend on to make herself clean. This emphasis on dislocation within the so-cial structure of village life recurred throughout the Fijian stories. In Fiji, it is the place and responsibility of the family to provide the needed care for all members. Failures to meet hygiene and other body norms signal a lack of love and concern within the rest of the family, mak-ing them all look bad by association.[19]

In the United States, Brittany described a woman who was very poor and so didn't have access to a shower. This could be because she was sick, unemployed, addicted to drugs, or mentally ill.

In New Zealand, Vicky created a rich backstory for the socially un-acceptable, unclean woman. Vicky told us she had a nasty divorce. The children wouldn't talk to her. Her life went the wrong way. She lost her job and couldn't pay the bills. She ended up "carrying a trolley" (that is, homeless and keeping her belongings in a shopping cart).[20]

Across all four sites, in our analysis of the full dataset, we found that hygiene norm violations were clearly *stigmatized* (table 2.2). They were associated with other stigmatized identities, like homelessness (figure 2.3), being unemployed, or being a very low-paid worker. Inter-estingly, across all the sites, these stigmatized identities carried eco-nomic stigma; that is, the women were socially devalued because of their low socioeconomic class or impoverished economic position.

What Is the Link between Hygiene Stigma and Waterborne Disease Risk?

To test the idea that hygiene stigma and infectious disease risk are closely related, we next coded respondents' statements to see if they raised illness, disease, or other health concerns in their discussions of

TABLE 2.2.
Thematic differences in cultural perceptions of hygiene in four global sites

Fiji	Guatemala	New Zealand	United States
Percentage of deaths due to lack of sanitation and hygiene[1]			
3.8%	8.1%	0%	0.4%
Blame burden			
Higher, but blame placed on the family	Lower, due to economic inequality, plight of the working poor	Higher, person mostly to blame due to bad choices	Moderate, mitigating circumstances like ill-fortune
Social identity of an unacceptably unclean woman			
Person without relatives, an outsider, "grog"/drug addict, mentally ill/crazy	Farm worker, low-paid worker, beggar, trash picker	Homeless, unemployed, dole bludger,[2] divorced	Drug addict, homeless, mentally ill
Common adjectives			
Unloved, uncaring of self, uneducated, outsider, old, disgusting	Poor, impoverished, lazy	Scary, creepy, mentally ill	Down on one's luck, abused, poor

1. "Mortality and Burden of Disease from Water and Sanitation," World Health Organization, August 29, 2018, http://www.who.int/gho/phe/water_sanitation/burden_text/en/.
2. A person who is able to work but pretends they can't in order to receive unemployment benefits from the government.

hygiene violations. Fiji, by far, had more indicators of ill-health mentioned alongside hygiene violations than the other three countries. The most commonly identified diseases were skin infections, especially scabies and ringworm. These itchy diseases, caught through prolonged close body contact, are relatively minor but common in Fiji. Beyond this, drug and alcohol use and abuse also emerged as part of the backstories of the unclean woman. In Fiji, interviewees mentioned the overuse of kava, or "grog," which is a ceremonial drink whose sedative properties are also enjoyed through bouts of communal recreational drinking. Mostly groups of men drink it together, so stories of a Fijian woman having too much kava suggests someone who is socially isolated and unaligned with Fijian customs.

In Guatemala, only four people mentioned disease markers or symptoms. One respondent said the socially unacceptable, unclean woman had "many illnesses." Another said the unclean woman was intellectually impaired. A third respondent said the unclean woman was a "drug addict," and a fourth said she was a "drunk." In Guatemala, where water scarcity and waterborne disease risk were highest among our sites, there were no specific signifiers of *infectious* disease at all. In New Zealand, the most common health indicator mentioned was mental health. Examples of such descriptors included "she might have mental issues," "mad person," "severe mental illness," "depressed," and "down and depressed." There was also mention of substance abuse problems described variously as "alcoholic," "drugs," "smoker," and "struggles with addiction."

In the United States, like New Zealand, descriptions of the socially unacceptable, unclean woman centered on mental health and substance abuse. Common statements included "a drug addict," "probably a drug dealer or prostitute," and "maybe a former drug abuser." Others thought the unclean woman might be "mentally ill" or have a "mental condition." Here, as in New Zealand, there was no mention at all of infectious disease.

Given the large amount of data we collected and the many ways we probed respondents, surprisingly little was said about disease—but enough was said to detect some basic patterns across the sites. In both the United States and New Zealand, explanations for why women might violate hygiene norms relied nearly exclusively on mental illness and/or substance abuse. In Fiji, too, substance abuse and mental illness emerged as themes, but skin diseases such as sores, scabies, and ringworm played a larger role in the narratives. In Guatemala, the site where we expected to find the tightest link between infectious disease and hygiene stigma, there were very few mentions of disease at all. In sum, our ethnographic evidence strongly indicates that respondents did *not* associate hygiene stigma with infectious disease.

Beyond these basic patterns, there was some variation across the sites in the way that social structure played into narratives about women's hygiene stigma. In Fiji, hygiene stigma was linked to being an outsider, being rejected by the family, or from the "other village." Moreover, when disease was mentioned, it was in relation to very minor skin infections, not anything that could do much real damage. In Guatemala, hygiene stigma was more linked to what academics might call structural poverty, or the barriers that prevent people from earning a living wage and removing themselves from poor living conditions. In New Zealand and the United States, responses attached hygiene stigma to an urban underclass who had fallen on hard luck due to divorce, unemployment, hard life circumstances, and drug problems or mental illness.

This all suggested to us that hygiene stigma is ultimately more about maintaining social status and boundaries, than it is about protecting people from infectious diseases. The notion that stigma is more about social inequalities and less about disease prevention is important in understanding the social damage stigma can do. This is the focus of our next chapter.

The Bottom Line

Based on the data we have collected, early anthropologist Mary Douglas was right. People everywhere attach local, socially devalued identities to those who violate local hygiene norms. But this stigmatization is not doing much to help people maintain a distance from disease contaminations, and people largely fail to make that connection. Instead, people consistently tie hygiene violations to social and economic marginalization. This underscores *why* stigma-based interventions in global health (like Community-Led Total Sanitation) will *always* carry the potential to do significant damage to the most vulnerable members of society.

3

Dirty and Disempowered

In Pain and in Debt in Appalachia

Tonya's front tooth is killing her.[1] Eating anything hot, sweet, chewy, or hard shoots intense waves of sharp pain up the side of her face. Living in a borrowed manufactured home at the end of an unpaved dead-end road in rural Virginia, United States, she is sticking to a diet of applesauce and milk until she can get it fixed. Down to her last seven, wobbling teeth in a mouth of red, inflamed gums, she maintains a careful daily routine of gently brushing and flossing despite the pain. She says the best thing would be to have all her remaining teeth pulled and dentures made. But there's no cash to pay a dentist. Her husband's chronic lung disease has pushed him into disability, halving the family income. She used to work as a part-time school bus driver. But now, like many of her neighbors in poverty-stricken central Appalachia, she is both unemployed and uninsured.

Worse, as she explained to anthropologist Sarah Raskin, Tonya knows her mouth looks like a "damned carved pumpkin." She rarely smiles because it is so humiliating. Her profound dental damage also means she isn't welcomed at the local hospital emergency room, where she could at least get some serious pain relief. The medical staff don't see a 47-year-old struggling mother in desperate need of their care. Her "bombed-out" mouth evokes those shocking health department anti-methamphetamine drug use posters. They signal a

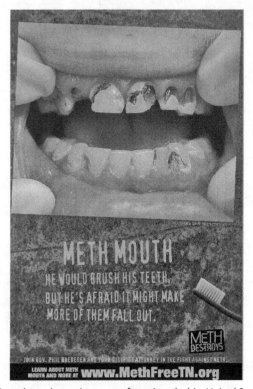

Figure 3.1. Anti-methamphetamine poster from Appalachia, United States. From Nexus Coalition for Drug Prevention

possible addict, using phantom tooth pain to extract a bottle of prescription opioids (figure 3.1).

To Tonya, her mouthful of decay reflects a lifetime of effort and brave suffering. But to others, it quickly stigmatizes her as an unworthy person. White, straight teeth and sweet breath are highly socially valued in the United States. Good teeth suggest a good person, one who has invested the expected time, effort, and money in self-care and regular dental visits. By contrast, her decayed, broken, and missing teeth conjure a long past of moral failings. Not just possible drug use, but perhaps improper or absent parenting, long lapses of poor personal hygiene, or an uncontrolled diet of sugar and junk food.[2] Bad teeth are also sometimes taken to suggest other deficits, like low intelligence, mental illness, homelessness, and poverty.[3]

But this ready judgment by hospital staff and others Tonya en-counters belies an obvious economic fact. Dentistry is mostly a pri-vate profession, and, in many countries, the mouth is one of the most expensive body parts to treat. Even in some of the wealthier nations like the United States, the costs of basic, regular preventive care stretch beyond easy affordability for many. In low- and middle-income coun-tries, it is completely out of reach for large sectors of society.[4] Perhaps it's no surprise then that between 60 and 90 percent of schoolchildren globally are walking around with untreated dental cavities in their mouths, making it the most common chronic childhood disease.[5] Having bad teeth doesn't make you a "bad" person; it more likely means you can't easily afford to visit a dentist.

A lifetime of denied access to regular preventive care cascades into oral catastrophes like Tonya's. And, for people who can barely afford dental prevention, emergency procedures are economic catastrophes too. Estimated globally, the cost of a single treatment is, on average, over 40 percent of family monthly budgets. As a result, millions of fam-ilies worldwide are pushed over the poverty line by getting their tooth pain fixed, forced to take loans they can't afford or forgo basic neces-sities like food and water.[6]

But add the discrimination that comes from the association be-tween bad teeth and bad people, and everything worsens.[7] Once her teeth were visibly decayed, this further eroded Tonya's chances to get dental or hospital care, a good job with dental insurance, or otherwise get out of her situation. Tonya's painful tooth exemplifies how easily damaging hygiene stigmas—like the assumption that good people have good teeth—are locked-in with poverty and with often inescap-able consequences to physical health.

Dirty and Depressed in Bolivia

This toxic combination of hygiene stigma and need doesn't just ex-aggerate physical and economic suffering. It devastates emotionally too, feeding self-doubt, worry, and distress in ways that even further undermine people's capacity to cope. When Amber first met Doña

Juana in 2003, she had been living in the dusty Bolivian informal settlement of Villa Israel on the margins of Cochabamba city for twenty years.[8] Always quick-witted and insightful, she and her husband worked night shifts to support their four children, and his mother and brother. Their neighborhood—painstakingly self-built homes, stores, and churches—was established on illegally subdivided land. After a long and costly fight for recognition from the municipality, Doña Juana knew city services like running water weren't coming to Villa Israel any time soon.

So, the community worked hard together to improve things as best they could. The year before, with support they had won from a government program, Doña Juana and other neighborhood women had worked to dig out stormwater channels. The women spent days hauling and stacking boulders to divert a river's course away from their homes during summertime flash floods that may endanger their children and cut their neighborhood off from jobs and schools in the city. Years previously, they had built their shared tap stand system to bring water closer to their homes, fed by pipe from a well in the hills above the settlement.

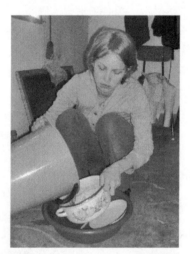

Figure 3.2. Amber washing dishes with limited water in Villa Israel, during fieldwork in Cochabamba, Bolivia, 2004. Photo by R. Aguilar and W. Valencia

As one of the first settlers in Villa Israel, Doña Juana remembered early days when there was enough water for growing corn and other crops in her own small garden. Now, with the community growing so fast, there wasn't enough water for even a quarter of the homes (figure 3.2). As a homeowner, Doña Juana knew she was one of the lucky ones, eligible to pay the monthly fee and wait in line each day for her allotted four buckets of water from the community water system.[9] This might be enough to drink, but Doña Juana constantly worried about how her family would flush the toilet, keep their home presentable, and wash themselves and their clothes. Without enough water to splash off the dust of the neighborhood, Doña Juana fretted that her children would be teased at school for having dirty faces and clothes.

When they had the money, one option was to buy more water from the large tanker trucks that passed through the neighborhood each day. This took effort because the drivers didn't like to stop for small purchases like hers, their arrival was unpredictable, and the water was expensive. Even if you could beg a driver to stop and fill your bucket, you had to endure their disdain at your poverty. Some days, her husband would have to take hours off work to search further afield for someone to sell them water. But worse, when all else failed, she was forced to beg her neighbors to sell her what little water they had. The experience was so painful that Doña Juana often found herself avoiding any contact with them for weeks after.

The constant struggle to get water took a heavy toll. The family argued often, seething under the constant stress. Doña Juana was always working, tired, and fighting back despair. Her family and house were not as clean as she thought they should be, because without water she couldn't get the dust out of the house or off their clothes. She felt constantly judged by others because she was dirty. She was chagrined by what she saw as her own failure to live up to the most basic expectations of sanitation, and so, decency.

Amber heard many similar stories, of the daily worry and humiliations around meeting social and hygienic expectations, from the seventy-two household heads that were in that 2004–2005 water

insecurity study in Cochabamba.[10] The household heads she interviewed were randomly selected from the total of 415 households Amber's team identified and mapped in the small community. Almost
three-quarters reported they had less than the five buckets (fifty
liters) of water per person for daily use, the minimum daily requirement for survival according to the World Health Organization. As clean
water ran out, families resorted to drinking contaminated water;[11]
nearly a quarter of households reported dehydration or intestinal illness (i.e., diarrhea) as a result.

And, the numbers showed, that profound stress around inadequate
and unsafe water is highly associated with the types of distress that
can be associated with depression and anxiety: 92 percent said they
had been fearful, 88 percent said they were worried, 79 percent reported they were angry over water issues within the prior week. But
it was those women who had to regularly plead neighbors for help
who had the most persistent signs of extreme emotional distress.
They were deeply humiliated that they had to beg for water. For some,
this emotional distress could become debilitating, making it hard to
accomplish even the basic social and economic functions like running
a household or getting or keeping a job. This is another example of
how living with hygiene stigma—the struggle to prove "I am a clean
and, therefore, a good person" even when you do not have the amenities available to do so—can push those in poverty down even further.

These women's struggles to manage the social consequences of living without water provides us a tiny glimpse at what is a constantly
unfolding, nearly invisible, global tragedy. Consider three key facts.
First, more than two billion households globally are struggling to get
enough safe water and shortages are increasing. Second, depression
is already one of the most common illnesses globally.[12] Third, encouraging better sanitation remains a main focus in global health efforts
and promoting the idea of cleanliness as a virtue is central to that. This
suggests that millions upon millions, all across the globe, are living
with the same anguish as Doña Juana: feeling distress that they aren't
"decent, worthy" people—just because they don't have enough water.
When considering water insecurity in places like Cochabamba as a

public health challenge to solve, it is easy to assume that having enough safe water to drink is where the problem ends. But, until we recognize how the effort to avoid hygiene stigma raises the stakes, five buckets of water a day is simply not enough to keep people healthy, mentally and physically.

Unsanitary and Undermined across South America

Hygiene stigmas aren't just a burden to individuals. They can easily adhere to whole groups of politically powerless people, triggering wider suffering in the form of epidemics. This is exactly what happened with the wave of deadly waterborne cholera that raced through South America in the early 1990s.[13] Cholera is a diarrheal disease that triggers stigmas of being "unclean" and "disgusting" easily, because it is transmitted by untreated human waste.

In August 1992, in Venezuela's remote, forested Mariusa delta region where the wide, brown Orinoco River meets the ocean, Santiago Rivera died (figure 3.3).[14] The middle-aged governor of a small indigenous Warao community, Santiago supported his family by pulling crabs from their holes in the muddy river floor. He had first doubled over with

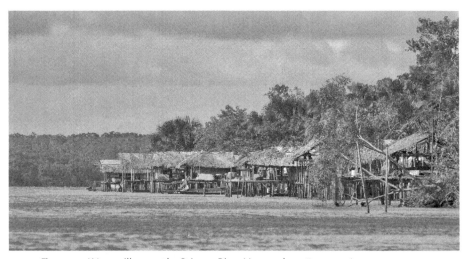

Figure 3.3. Warao village on the Orinoco River, Venezuela. © Shutterstock

painful abdominal cramps on a foraging trip to gather palm starch with his sister and wife. Then came the explosive diarrhea and vomiting. The family immediately suspected malicious magic was the cause. An enemy of Santiago's had crossed their path in the rainforest that day. But none of the local curers' songs, massages, or herbs worked, and Santiago passed shortly after. Seven more people in their village died with the same symptoms in the next four days. In such a small place—where everyone was related in some fashion—the new and mysterious spreading illness was creating confusion, panic, and terror.

When public health officials at the regional head office in Tucupita were alerted about the deaths in Mariusa, they immediately recognized cholera. Transmitted through infected sewage entering drinking water supplies or contaminating shellfish, it is extremely contagious. Death by dehydration can happen within hours. But cholera is also easy to identify and responds well to antibiotic treatment and simple efforts at rehydration. This means public health is well-equipped to easily and cheaply treat it—if caught soon enough. No one needs to die. They knew the key was educating the public and medical staff in how to recognize the signs and letting them know they had to then move quickly. So, they did one round of training for medical staff in the large central town. Further, they provided information in the local newspaper to residents so they would know to treat their drinking water with bleach to make it safe and to rush to the hospital at the first sign of profuse, watery diarrhea.

But for the forty thousand Warao who lived rurally in the delta around Santiago Rivera's community, none of this happened. Too far from the cities and with little economic or political power, they were already underserved by the country's medical and public health infrastructure. Many families also lacked any practical means for a safe water supply or the money to buy soap or toilet paper. The Warao, those most at risk of contracting cholera, were never provided with this key information that could have helped them prepare themselves for the rapid spread of the disease that followed.

This was because they were already stigmatized by those in the cities as dirty, disgusting, unsanitary people. As the epidemic unfolded, public health officer press statements were quick to highlight their ignorance. They explained how they didn't want to use toilets or want to wash their hands and didn't understand how to use toilet paper. Their accounts never acknowledged how the lack of facilities or medical services in the delta might be responsible, nor that someone from the outside must have brought in the disease to the Warao (likely a passing commercial fisherman from a large city to the southwest). Authorities, from the president on down, even initially chalked the outbreak up to the "normal" types of diarrhea that inevitably hit "filthy" indigenous people.

This official narrative, that the problem was dirty people not dirty water, made those in the larger towns and cities feel safe from what was happening to the Warao. But this calming version of the growing calamity also meant the public health response was slow and lackluster in the rural areas of the delta. Minimal medical staff and supplies were dispatched and only with delay. And so, the epidemic spread, killing hundreds that could have been saved by an earlier, more aggressive, and more appropriate public health response.

By early 1993, the epidemic had spread to the cities of northeastern Brazil. There, too, cholera was an intimate ally of poverty and powerlessness, particularly striking the massive favelas (impoverished urban communities). The same dangerous pattern of blaming these "disgusting" *favelados* for their lack of sanitation repeated itself. But this time, the people living in the favelas pushed back against the stigma and shame assigned to them by public health workers. And, when this happened, the epidemic spread even faster.

The 440 families—that crowded in their small, self-built, stick-and-mud homes along Avenida Gonçalves Dias in Brazil's coastal Fortaleza city—had no city water or sewerage services.[15] Raw waste was thrown out from the tightly packed homes into the gutters. And they certainly didn't have desperately needed public amenities. They had already been expelled by the city four times as unwanted residents in recent years. Medical researchers from the local university expected the incoming cholera epidemic would hit these families hard. They had been tracking diarrheal disease on the Avenida for several years

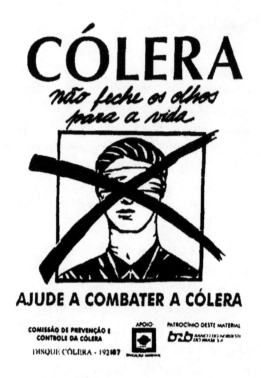

CÓLERA
não feche os olhos para a vida

AJUDE A COMBATER A CÓLERA

COMISSÃO DE PREVENÇÃO E
CONTROLE DA CÓLERA
DISQUE CÓLERA - 192187

APOIO·

PATROCÍNIO DESTE MATERIAL

Figure 3.4. Anti-cholera poster, Venezuela, 1993, reads "don't close your eyes to life." Reproduced from M. K. Nations and C. M.G. Monte, "'I'm Not Dog, no!': Cries of Resistance against Cholera Control Campaigns," *Social Science & Medicine* 43, no. 6 (1996): 1007–1024

and knew it was already the main cause of the many child deaths there.

Traditional healer and Avenida resident Dona Zilnar had already herself lost several children to diarrheal illnesses. But when a community health worker handed her the note confirming the lab identification of *Vibrio cholera* from her stool sample, she responded unexpectedly: "Here, we don't have cholera, no!" she spat. "Somebody invented it, and they are going to invent more to come!" Balling up the paper and throwing it to the ground she yelled: "What do you think I am, some low-down, stray mutt dog?" She didn't want any of their treatment. She suspected this talk of cholera was probably some form of con, devised to take advantage of the poor and once again displace them from their housing.

The Avenida's residents had heard the announcements on the radio, warning about the rising epidemic. They understood the implications behind all the talk about the squalid conditions that created cholera—neighborhoods with open sewers and children playing in the streets without shoes. They knew these reports were describing places like the Avenida. It meant *they* were filthy and disgusting, like stray dogs in the street. The national cholera campaign slogan, "Get out cholera!" sounded to them like "Get out, you worthless, cholera-infected person."

The official campaign posters portrayed a blindfolded man with a giant red X slashed across his face (figure 3.4). The image of the poster suggested the cholera-infected were marked to die, political pawns in a larger conspiracy. To the residents of Avenida, the war against cholera was a war on them. *They* were the cholera that threatened everyone else, most especially the city's elite. They responded as best they knew how. Suspecting they were being poisoned, they began spitting out antibiotic pills and tossing away the bleach. Fearing they may be rounded up, they misled health workers as to who was sick, avoided diagnostic tests, and refused hospital care.

Denied real political power to challenge their living conditions or respond to their everyday stigma as "disgusting" people, the Avenida's residents fought back in the only way they could: They denied the disease itself. A culture of blaming the poor for their own plight and labeling them as dirty had backfired badly. It had completely eroded even the most basic community trust in public health institutions. The result was cholera hitting higher-income parts of the city too. The disease roared in Brazil because the people of the favelas were given no voice.

Nearly three decades later, we saw exactly the same deadly game—of shifting the blame of cholera down onto the poorest and least powerful—unfold all over again. Haiti has been in the grip of a new cholera epidemic since 2010. It arrived from Nepal in the intestines of United Nations (UN) peacekeepers, there to provide assistance in the wake of a devastating earthquake. The bacteria leaked from poorly treated sewage at the UN camp into the Artibonite River, snaking through

Haiti and along the border of the Dominican Republic. The UN was very slow to respond with even a declaration of responsibility, let alone any major, concrete assistance to prevent further deaths.[16]

In a low-income country dealing with a serious and costly natural disaster, Haitian public health and water infrastructures were utterly inadequate to manage a cholera outbreak (figure 3.5). When we did community-based interviews there in 2017, the epidemic was still in full swing. Nearly ten thousand Haitians were dead and nearer to a million had been sickened. But, when we talked with people in the most underserved communities where many households often ran out of food and water, they didn't blame the cholera deaths on the UN or their own government. They said the cause was simply dirty water.[17]

But as the epidemic started to seep into the waterways of the wealthier Dominican Republic next door, the blame took on a different shape.[18] It wasn't dirty water spreading disease, people said, but the "dirty Haitian" migrant workers. Accordingly, the Dominican authorities were not inclined to help. Instead, many blamed Haitian migrant workers—most living without basic services, healthcare, and with dreadful discrimination—for their misfortune. This predictable downhill flow of stigma onto those who are most vulnerable nearly always accelerates disease epidemics.

In both of these major waves of cholera—in the 1990s in South America and more recently in Haiti—we are able also to see how the stigma toward "disgusting" people living without basic sanitation is embedded within political and healthcare institutions, both large and small. And, over and over, this undermines the capacity of these institutions to help the very people that most need it. This begs the question: Why does this same pattern keep repeating, even though it is clear the stigma is feeding the very epidemics it seeks to vanquish? The answer is because declaring people "unsanitary subjects"— disgusting, diseased, and dangerous—has power.[19] Sometimes the gains might be small (if valuable), like when the authorities in Venezuela were able to reassure the majority of their worried voters that

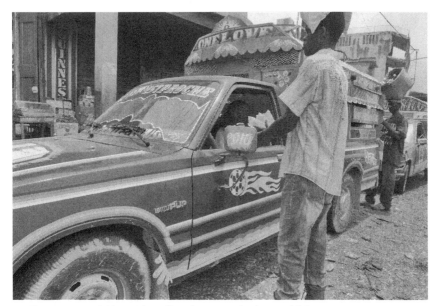

Figure 3.5. Roadside vendor selling clean water by the pouchful to "tap tap" passengers in Port-au-Prince, Haiti. © Shutterstock

they were still safe despite the cholera outbreak on the delta. Other times the benefits could be very large. One benefit could be, for instance, gaining valuable land for urban development in Brazil. Another benefit could be saving the millions of dollars it would cost to provide adequate water infrastructure for all Haitians. The same scenario repeats again and again because someone is benefitting.

Diseased and Deposed in Hawai'i

Dona Zilner suspected a grand conspiracy against the people like her, struggling on the margins of society. And sometimes, there actually is one. History shows that applying hygiene stigmas to whole groups can prove to be an especially potent force for consolidating power. By tapping into people's deep-seated fears of contagion, gains can be as great as entire countries. This is exactly what happened in Hawai'i in the second half of the nineteenth century.

In 1882, young cowboy Kaluaikoʻolau spent his days working in the mountains of the lush Hawaiʻian island of Kauaʻi, wrangling cattle with his rawhide rope and hunting with his rifle.[20] Life was certainly not easy for Hawaiʻians at the time. Deathly epidemics new to the islands, like measles and smallpox, were raging. With no acquired immunity, these diseases had been decimating the Hawaiʻian population.

Yet Kaluaikoʻolau himself was happy and had good reason for optimism. The previous year he had married his childhood sweetheart Piʻilani in the church at Waimea. His joy was now compounded with the birth of a strong son, Kaleimanu (figure 3.6). But life complicated for the young family in 1889, when Kaluaikoʻolau noticed a strange rash on his cheek. At first, the couple thought perhaps it was a reaction to the sun or to soap. But then similar rashes appeared on their son's body. They realized, with growing dread, these were likely the early signs of leprosy.[21] They were terrified and kept it to themselves.

The family's terror wasn't due to a fear of the disease itself. Hawaiʻians, unlike Europeans, didn't fear or stigmatize the disease at all. They were happy to eat with, sleep with, and care for those infected.[22] Rather, the family's fear was based on what happened after the telltale rashes and scars of the bacterial infection were discovered by the authorities. The European and American settlers that were descending on the Hawaiʻian islands had been declaring people with leprosy as morally "unclean" since the Middle Ages.[23] And the authorities were quick to quarantine Hawaiʻians with leprosy. It was the reason Hawaiʻians sometimes referred to leprosy as *mai hoʻokaʻawale*, the separating sickness.

In 1865, the newly formed Hawaiʻian Public Health Board had passed their "Act to Prevent the Spread of Leprosy," mandating quarantine for those identified with the disease.[24] The board selected and purchased the distant, isolated Kalaupapa peninsula on the island of Molokaʻi for the purpose. The highest sea cliffs in the world provided a formidable physical barrier, only reached by a single steep trail with twenty-six switchbacks covering a drop of 1,700 vertical feet. Who went and who didn't was determined by the government. In the years that followed, some eight thousand native Hawaiʻians were shipped

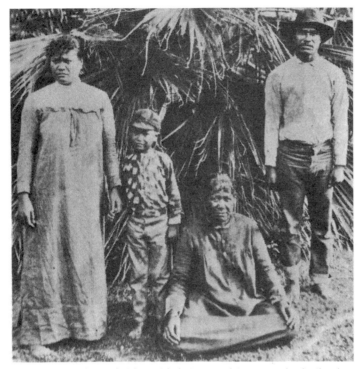

Figure 3.6. Kaluaikoʻolau and Piʻilani with their son, Kaleimanu, and Kaluaikoʻolau's mother, Kukui Kaleimanu. From the Hawaii State Archives

to the new leper colony, most torn away from their families against their will. They called Kalaupapa "the grave where one is buried alive."

As the young family had feared, Kaluaikoʻolau's facial marks were noticed one day in the market. The government doctor declared him sick and slated him for transfer by ship to Molokaʻi. But the rest of the family were to stay behind. Desperate to be together, they packed their horses and rode for a remote valley. For the next several months, Piʻilani and Kaluaikoʻolau quietly gardened and foraged a living from the cool, rainy mountainside, banded together in a small community with other leprosy refugees.

One clear midmorning in 1893, right after the overthrow of the Hawaiʻian monarchy, Deputy High Sheriff Louis Stoltz rode in from the town of Waimea. The board of health was rounding up those slated for quarantine for transport to Molokaʻi. Anticipating resistance because the families were being wrenched apart, armed police were dispatched. In the ensuing melee, Kaluaikoʻolau shot the sheriff and another officer. The family hastily retreated into the thick bush in the remote reaches of the valley. The president of the health board himself, William Owen Smith, sailed in from Honolulu to help with the hunt for the resisters, with more army soldiers and three coffins in tow. But the family was never captured, and they stayed lost for the next four years. Once her son and then husband weakened and died from complications of malnutrition and leprosy, Piʻilani walked out to tell their story.

Kaluaikoʻolau's death is wrapped within a larger tale, one with all the hallmarks of grand conspiracy. The Public Health Board was more effective at solidifying control of the islands than dealing with the decimation of the indigenous Hawaiʻian population by infectious disease. The board that criminalized so many Hawaiʻians for their leprosy was comprised of the sons of missionaries and businessmen from the United States. They saw fortunes to be made by turning large tracts of land into the cane plantations that could produce sugar for the rapidly growing US market. But control of Hawaiʻian land required the full dismantling of the Hawaiʻian monarchy's power.

The health board fully embraced the notion that Hawaiʻians were getting sick and dying because they were unsanitary and otherwise constitutionally weak. The notion that Hawaiʻians were especially susceptible to leprosy also bolstered the argument that their queen was unfit to rule. This was of great use to their close friends on the thirteen-member "safety committee" that later engineered her removal—with the help of the US military. It also reinforced the idea that the islands would inevitably lose self-rule anyway and would be much better managed by (white) Americans. By leveraging fear around and stigma toward leprosy, they also made sure that Kaluaikoʻolau and anyone else displaying any form of resistance to the new government were portrayed as dangerous.

Quarantine, thus, proved itself a highly effective means to maintain political control following the fall of the monarchy, right as native Hawaiʻians began organizing for Queen Liliʻuokalani's restoration. Those high sea cliffs were not just about public sanitation, they were in many ways a political prison too. But it was the stigma that was foisted on the Hawai'ians as unclean,[25] dangerous lepers that made those cruel, lifelong internments seem somehow right, proper, valid, and justified.[26] In 1895, the Kingdom of Hawai'i was formally dissolved. Two years later, the US government successfully annexed the islands. Hygiene stigma had been deployed to great political advantage, quelling Hawai'ian resistance and benefiting the new American leaders with control of the islands and what would become highly profitable plantations.[27]

The Bottom Line

The struggles of Tonya, Doña Juana, Santiago Rivera, Dona Zilnar, and Kaluaiko'olau are all cautionary tales about how labeling people as dirty and disgusting creates more illness and suffering. Dental disease worsens. Depression sets in. Epidemics flare. Livelihoods are ruined. Families are wrenched apart. People who are powerless and in poverty, those typically denied adequate sanitation to begin with, then become even more so.

But, together, these stories—spanning two centuries and the entire globe—pull into focus a bigger picture. Hygiene stigma is very damaging because it connects to our core emotions and is then easily projected onto whole groups. By defining those with less power as unsanitary, hygiene stigmas can be all-too-easily deployed for the political and economic gain by those who already have it.[28]

This is why any form of sanitation intervention in poor and otherwise marginalized communities—from teaching dental hygiene to responding to outbreaks of waterborne disease—needs to take heed of Dona Zilner's suspicions. Constant vigilance is required to recognize public health efforts that blame, shame, and stigmatize people who are seen as "dirty." Without this, the best-intentioned efforts can quickly cause damage, distance, and disempowerment. In doing so, they can undermine the ideals of global health as a major force for creating health, reducing poverty, and advancing social justice.

Part II

Lazy

Fat, Bad, and Everywhere

Fat.[1] It's a very powerful word—one loaded with failure, blame, and shame. It's common to hear comments suggesting fat people are lazy and ignorant, have no self-respect or self-control, or are less lovable. Even the medical term for excess weight, "obesity," implies an impending doom and disaster. It's cast as a deadly epidemic caused by fat people's bad choices. They are solely responsible for their own plight. From policy makers to media, from families and friends to strangers on the street, everyone agrees on one thing: Fat is bad. But it seems our fear of excess weight has evolved into a disgust for the those who have it. Our collective public health efforts to fight fat often feel like a campaign against fat people themselves.[2] The message to each of us is clear: to be normal, to be acceptable, to be healthy, *you* must take control. Stop being lazy.

These moralizing views of fat are everywhere, and they permit systematic and serious discrimination. Solid data from studies in the United States, the United Kingdom, and Western Europe show when body fat goes up, wages go down, no matter how well they do their job or how well-educated they are.[3] People who are the largest have the hardest time landing a job, more trouble getting accepted into college, less chance of getting promoted, and greater risk of being fired. The stigma of living with extreme weight is not just an emotional struggle; it is a physical struggle too. Just consider flying. Airline seats have shrunken considerably over the last decade. Many provide just 16.5 inches for each passenger to sit in. This is not a comfortable or adequate size for one-third or more of adults from places as diverse as Australia, Samoa, and the United Arab Emirates. And for people who are especially large, those categorized as morbidly obese,[4] getting up to the use the tiny airline bathroom is a particularly difficult physical challenge. To add to the humiliation and punishment further, if you are too big to fit in a "normal"-sized seat, airlines will make you pay extra for a second one. The entire experience seems designed to constantly remind that you don't belong out in public society. This example shows why weight stigma has been called the last socially acceptable discrimination.[5] The result: People suffer their whole lives through chronic, all-consuming efforts to shed both weight and the dreadful shame, social rejection, and physical discomfort that it carries.

This severe anti-fat bias seeps into many other unexpected aspects of modern daily life, too,[6] most of it unconsciously. Juries are more likely to convict someone who is fatter, independent of the details of the crime.[7] Fat people are seen to be less trustworthy. Parents pay less college tuition for overweight daughters,[8] because they are viewed as a less promising investment. People are less willing to date someone larger. Fat people aren't considered as sexy, or if someone slimmer prefers to date them, it might be called a fetish. Larger children are teased, bullied, and left out. They aren't desirable as friends, and they somehow seem easy, acceptable fodder for schoolyard humiliation.[9] Parents of larger children are blamed too, considered the neglectful cause for their children's unacceptable size. Some have even had their children taken away.[10]

The casualness of everyday weight stigma also means that it is barely seen for what it is. Giggling at "fatties" on television and sizing them out of booths at restaurants feels "natural"—how things are and how they should be. It's so taken for granted that even an elementary school book designed to increase empathy toward overweight children has a subtly fat-shaming cover. More overtly, the text inside declares that stupidity and ignorance are the real cause of weight gain. It offers advice like "[fat kids] need someone like their friends or family or teachers to learn how to take care of themselves by eating less and exercising more."[11] In other words, it's fat kids' problem to fix themselves.

Excess, unhealthy body weight is absolutely an important public health challenge to be addressed. It triggers health-destructive, metabolic changes like uncontrolled blood sugar and hardening arteries. Sufficient, sustained weight loss can often fix chronic, expensive-to-treat diseases like diabetes without medication, reduce disability, and add years to people's lives. But this entire approach often assumes that people (even kids) can lose weight easily if they just *apply* themselves. However, study upon study shows that dropping weight permanently (especially once you are technically obese) is really, really hard.

There is not a new worldwide epidemic of laziness; obesity rates are skyrocketing because of changing food and exercise environments. Take for example the fact that you need a car to get to your office, where you then sit all day at a computer screen. The solutions to changing societal patterns such as these must be much bigger than any individual losing weight. We need thoughtful, public transportation systems within walking distance and redesigned office spaces with walking desks. But that's not the public message being delivered about why people are getting bigger. Instead, the message we're giving and getting is putting the blame elsewhere: It's *your* fault.

The public would rather pay for treatments for cigarette addiction than for preventing weight gain or, especially, supporting weight loss.[12] Being fat is less excusable, it seems, than being a pack-a-day smoker. Perhaps it is no surprise then that those struggling with weight issues are likely to self-stigmatize, to believe their treatment is justified because it stems from their own inexcusable failure to control what they eat. When you are fat in a fat-hating society, the scales don't just measure your weight. They measure your worth. People see your fat first, and many can't look beyond it. They assume because you are big that you are lazy, stupid, lacking self-control, and unworthy of love. Strangers stare and snicker. Family members offer unsympathetic and unwanted diet advice. Doctors ignore what you try to tell them, assuming any medical problem you have must be because of your weight. Even in the most advanced healthcare systems—right under our highly educated and informed noses—blaming people for their fat is utterly embedded in every aspect of how we treat them. This mistreatment is mostly perfectly legal and socially tolerated.

And it hurts emotionally. In our several decades of studying the social dimensions of obesity, we have heard the same distressed message expressed in many different ways, by many different people, and in many different languages. Karin Kwambai, writing of her lifetime struggle with her weight explains

> I am obese. That phrase is actually very hard for me to say out loud. Saying it feels as if I am standing at an "obesity anonymous" meeting, except there is nothing anonymous about being fat. Everyone knows it. I often feel that it is the first and only thing people notice about me. I've been overweight, chubby, fat my entire life. My mom enrolled me in Weight Watchers when I was 12 years old . . . I've learned a lot of maladjusted behaviors around food over a lifetime of trying to lose weight. I've tried meal replacement shakes, pills, souping, juicing, and the "Master Cleanse" . . . All of these tactics only messed up my mind and body even more. The summer before my freshman year of college, I literally ate only an apple a day because I was so worried about not making new friends because of my weight. It was not about being healthy; it was about being accepted. Following medical advice works until it stops working, and the weight comes back—plus some.[13]

This desperation to find any solution, however unhealthy, is understandable given the really nasty things people say, openly, when it comes to fat. In 2011, our cross-cultural research on weight stigma was featured on the front page of the *New York Times* (NYT). It generated a mass of online comments,[14] many of which were deeply hateful. The NYT broke their own policy and left this hateful trolling online. The writer that we worked with explained their decision in an email to us that said, "The people who post negative comments about larger people are simply proving the point of the story—that bias and stigma against overweight people is pervasive and damaging." Yes, even the NYT's educated, worldly readership thinks being nasty to "fatties" is just fine. Consider the comment from Muriel in London that generated 337 approving "likes" from other readers:

> About time. Fat people shouldn't complain when they're given a dose of reality—that they spill onto other people's seats, drive health costs for everyone sky high and, in the case of obese women, even endanger their own unborn babies. They seem to be complaining that selfishness is not regarded as admirable.

Of course, some readers were just as surprised and horrified as the NYT writer, like a commenter naming themselves Barbara from Virginia, who wrote, "This thread has to be one of the saddest and most vicious I have ever read. Too many comments show no understanding or encouragement, just judgment."

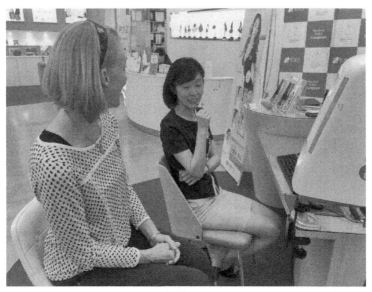

Figure 4.1. Conducting participant observation in hyper thin-obsessed Seoul, linguist Cindi SturtzSreetharan being talked through possible cosmetic surgeries, June 2016. Photo by A. Brewis

This "fat equals bad" thinking is already in full-force across all high-income nations. Two such places we have studied recently, South Korea and Norway, are vastly different in their cultural histories and current lifestyles. However, they illustrate how dramatically core beliefs about fat have globalized and converged. In 2015, the Oslo-based Center for Advanced Studies hosted Alex for a delightful summer of research and writing on the social dimensions of food. Fitness-obsessed Norway is a particularly fat-judgmental place, where excess weight is not tolerated.[15] It wasn't hard to find examples. The new Norwegian prime minister at the time, Erna Solberg, was heavily fat shamed in the press and on social media. Newspaper photos zoomed in on the candy package she bought to share with her cabinet. They featured humiliating shots of her bouncing on a trampoline. Norwegian social media chided, "It must be difficult to think when the woman is 99.9 percent fat with just a head on top for decoration."

Solberg went on Norwegian television to confront her trolls. She read this and other online comments out loud. Her summary message to help others cope with the shaming? You need a thick skin if you want to be in the public eye.[16] Self-stigma around fat is so pernicious and rampant that even one of the most successful women in the world saw herself as responsible for both the problem and the solution to being fat.

The following summer, we headed off to bustling Seoul with linguist Cindi SturtzSreetharan (figure 4.1) and demographer SeungYong Han to learn more about what people were saying and doing about weight in what we expected to be an especially stark case: Among the higher-income countries, South Korea has the very lowest obesity rates, in the order of 4–6 percent of adults. And, it is one of the most anti-fat societies in the world.[17] Cosmetic surgery rates there are, by far, the highest globally.

We visited South Korean schools, interviewed plastic surgeons, hung out at public bathhouses, lunched in private homes, and ventured onto soap opera sets. It quickly became clear that anti-fat messages and anxieties were everywhere. People would tell each other straight out, "I haven't seen you in a while, and—wow—you've got fatter." A colleague's mother told Alex, in a kind voice, "You are not fat . . . for an American."

South Koreans know their preferences for thinness, and concerns toward fat, are extreme. As we sat with colleagues at the Korean Women's Development Institute working through new research ideas, they galvanized when we demonstrated snippets of "fat talk," self-disparaging conversations where people connect to and get reassurances from others that they are not fat and thus they are okay.[18] Yes, they said, we do that all the time.

After the trip, we spent some time analyzing Korean national-level data to test some of the theories Korean experts and lay people suggested to us about the effects of fervent anti-fatness on other aspects of health.[19] Adults of all body sizes were really worried about being overweight. We found that efforts at weight loss were widely practiced among those who were ostensibly slim, even technically underweight. For women and men, overweight and underweight alike, displaying high levels of concern over the need to lose weight predicted a much higher risk of depression. As people's income and education increased, the effect just got worse.[20] And, in the context of a very unstable and competitive labor market in South Korea, those currently with steady employment seemed the most stressed about becoming or staying slim, engaging in potentially unhealthy weight-loss behaviors like taking pills and skipping meals.

Globalizing Fat Stigma

Despite this rampant, global, fat stigma today, the anthropological record is replete with examples from many societies of body fat being viewed as a *good* thing. In fact, the Human Relations Area Files (HRAF)[21] suggest that the majority (81 percent) of human societies historically have preferred plump bodies.[22] In many societies, large body size reflects moral virtue rather than failing. It means power, fertility, or plenty. Poor people are thin, while plump people are powerful and desirable. Rulers and leaders are fat.

One of the most detailed modern ethnographies that explains how fat is viewed as good is anthropologist Rebecca Popenoe's study with semi-nomadic Azawagh Arabs (Tuareg) in Saharan Africa.[23] She spent 1991 documenting how girls are force-fed to fatten their bodies into extreme beauty. Sitting immobile in the corners of tents, girls are goaded to drink buckets of camel's milk and eat mounds of porridge every day. The ample rolls of fat that resulted reflected their hard work and closeness to god. They also helped attract a good husband.

That very same year, Alex was doing long-term fieldwork on the opposite side of the globe. She was interviewing women about fertility and child-rearing on a small atoll in the Republic of Kiribati on the Pacific equator. Women there didn't purposefully fatten girls like the Tuareg did, but they did consider large bodies to be good bodies, and that skinny bodies needed to be fattened up. Bigger bodies were strong and could do important work, like gardening and feeding babies. Alex was subject to constant comments about being too skinny— having "legs you could see through." People would insist she ate

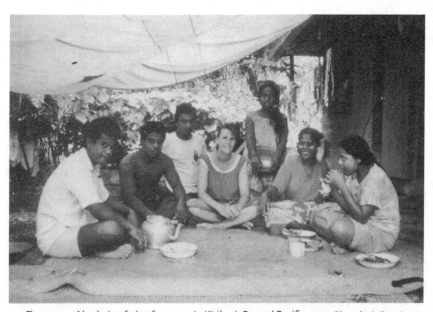

Figure 4.2. Alex being fed to fatten up in Kiribati, Central Pacific, 1990. Photo by A. Brewis

mountains of cold, white rice with dinner so she would plump up—and snag a good husband (figure 4.2).

A couple years later (1993–1995), Alex was doing fieldwork in nearby Samoa, where obesity rates had been high for some years. Large and strong bodies in Samoa had long been viewed as chiefly and powerful, but recently new ideas about the value of slimness had started to creep in. All the eighty-four women Alex interviewed (and most of them were very large) said they would like to be thinner than they were. Many of them had high body mass indexes, with the average body being in the "obese" category (BMI of 34.0). Their responses around weight concerns and need for weight loss were not that different than Samoan women living in New Zealand. For example, more than half of the women in both locations (56 percent and 66 percent respectively) had made some efforts to lose weight within the prior year. The main differences between the two sites was that Samoan women in New Zealand wanted to lose more weight and felt more compelled to do so even though they had lower body weights. In Samoa, women noted that losing weight didn't *really* matter to them—as people said they were fine as they were even if it would be a good thing for their health to lose some weight.[24] Thin idealism and worries around the medical issues weight created had both started to influence how people saw their bodies, but being fat was still okay too.[25]

Fast-forward another six years (2001), and Alex was doing research with middle-class, middle-school children in urban Mexico.[26] Much to her surprise, she discovered that many of these children were technically overweight or obese. In the sample of 219 children she measured, 24.9 percent were classifiable as overweight. The team spent several months observing kids at school; interviewing them, their parents, and classmates on standard psychometric scales and in one-on-one, open-ended interviews; and following them around during recess (a technique called "focal follows") to see what they were doing and who they hung out with. It turned out, statistically, that heavy children reported no greater experiences or feelings of stigma. They had similarly high self-esteem and the same risk of anxiety or depression as other children based on the standard scale measures. Importantly too, their classroom peers rated them no better or worse as friends. Basically, the data showed that body size didn't matter in their lives at all. And the doctors we talked with weren't worried either. They saw hungry, underfed children all the time, especially from the many informal settlements spread throughout the city. At that point, the value of the Mexican peso had collapsed, middle-class incomes were in freefall, and food insecurity was rife at the bottom of the socioeconomic ladder. Much better to be fat than thin, they explained.

Neoliberalism and Neo-norms

But a lot was changing in the 1990s and early 2000s. Perceptions of bigger bodies were starting to change in many places, including Mexico, Samoa, and Kiribati. Neoliberalism was spreading rapidly, and with it, new thinking about bodies and health that valorized individualism and self-responsibility.[27] New digital technologies also enabled faster and wider dissemination of stories and pictures of thin models and movie stars. As more countries adopted the cash economy, there were major changes in food production and more sedentary working lives. As a result, obesity rates were also rising sharply. For example, in Samoa, people were shifting from farming and fishing to less active jobs in tourism or factory work. Television and then the internet arrived, bringing new images of slimmer (and often utterly unattainable) bodies into people's daily lives.

By 2009, we had started to wonder what these new, powerful trends might mean for how people in historically fat-positive societies viewed big bodies. Our plan was to conduct a modest, exploratory study to map people's positive and negative attitudes toward obesity in ten countries around the world.[28] We included sites in places that we knew were historically fat-positive such as American Samoa, Mexico, Puerto Rico, and Tanzania. We also included, for comparison, some sites we considered likely to exhibit strong, anti-fat attitudes, like the upscale spa and golf vacation city of Scottsdale, Arizona, United States; London, England; and Buenos Aires, Argentina. We also threw in some wildcards to add more cultural diversity, like sites in New Zealand,

Iceland, and Paraguay, because there wasn't enough literature to know what to expect. In each place, we asked people whether they agreed or disagreed with the same list of statements, such as, "People are overweight because they are lazy." The results really surprised us. We found high levels of fat stigma in *all* of the ten countries we surveyed. Tanzanians scored an average of 10.4 (the least fat-negative of the sites surveyed), American undergraduates were at 12, and Paraguay were the very highest at 15 on the scale we developed.

In the years since we published this first, ten-country, cross-cultural study showing how common weight stigma was around the globe, many other anthropologists have confirmed the same basic finding. Fat stigma has been culturally adopted in many historically fat-positive places like India, Bolivia, and Dominica.[29] Unfortunately, we also see signs of a new global wave of discrimination in its wake. Take airline policies as an example. An Indian high court recently ruled that Air India, a state-owned enterprise, could refuse to employ overweight cabin staff. Similarly, Samoa Air has introduced a pay-by-weight system for domestic travelers. Weight itself has now become globally negative. Moreover, as incomes and education go up in low- and middle-income countries, this fat hate only seems to be getting stronger.

When we did our initial cross-cultural interviews in 2009, we were surprised to find that the small country of Paraguay popped up with the highest scores for explicit fat stigma—agreeing, for example, with the statement that "obese people should be ashamed of their bodies." Intrigued, we went back to Paraguay—where Amber has family and conducts fieldwork most summers—the following year to try to figure out why.

This time, we used implicit association tests (IATs) to assess fat stigma in Paraguay's capital city of Asuncion. Psychologists believe that IATs do a better job of capturing deep-seated, practiced prejudice. IATs are reaction-time tests that determine how quickly people connect the idea of fat to the idea of "bad" versus the idea of "good." The more experienced people are at thinking something, the faster they should be able to make connections. Essentially, IATs are designed to capture "what people think" about biases they may be unwilling or unable to admit.

Amazingly, we found that Paraguayan reaction time for "fat is good" and "fat is bad" were identical. This means that when Paraguayans insult someone else's weight, they are saying "fat is bad," but they are thinking "fat is fine." In other words, they are stating aloud the culturally, fat stigmatizing view, but they don't really mean it. The idea of "fat is bad" in Paraguay is *not* deeply internalized. Incidentally, this is *exactly* what people in Paraguay told us, but—as we learned in our other sites—you can't always take what people tell you about fat stigma at face value.

Our findings in Paraguay were very different from what we observed in places like the United States, United Kingdom, and New Zealand. There, people often talked "fat is fine" but thought "fat is bad." In these countries, IATs typically showed very high rates of implicit anti-fat thinking, often much higher than people would admit to when asked directly. For example, the American undergraduates we tested yielded an average IAT fat-negative score of 12, compared to 2.6 in Chennai, India, and 0.03 in Paraguay. At the same time, on self-reported questionnaires, anti-fat bias scores were much the same across the sites (64.6, 63.1, and 55.6 respectively, where higher scores indicate that people are *less* stigmatizing).[30]

At the same time though, people in all these countries will rarely insult someone's weight to their face. This apparent contradiction occurs because of a cultural rule that people are expected to suppress their prejudiced ideas in public. Psychologists call this a *justification-suppression* of prejudice.[31] American students we interviewed were doing just this. Paraguayans in our study were doing the exact opposite: expressing a prejudice on the surface that didn't seem to be held as a core belief deep down.

It's Complicated

Ethnographic research is arguably the best way to sort through these types of cultural incongruities. Paraguay is a place Amber knows very well. She has a second home and a vast network of beloved in-laws there. And of course, every time she visits, people comment on her weight and let her know exactly what they think about it. The data for Paraguay shows that rates of being overweight are very high (around 60 percent), while the rates of obesity are very low.[32] However, thin-idealizing body norms are everywhere. Walking down any city street, you see billboards, posters, and corner stores with images of scantily clad, thin-waisted women with well-endowed breasts and buttocks.

Amber spent the summer of 2017 doing more detailed, one-on-one interviews with Paraguayan women. She found them all highly conflicted about weight gain. It wasn't unusual to hear people say "wow, you got fat" or to make a fat joke, and a booming industry of nutritionists prescribe diet plans and sell diet foods to urbanites worried about their weight. At the same time, Paraguayans pride themselves on not having the extreme body norms and weight discrimination that they consider typical of neighboring Brazil and Argentina. Paraguay's "Miss Gordita" beauty pageant typifies these contradictions. The pageant crowns an ambassador to speak out against fat discrimination, even as pageant contestants are asked for advice on how others can lose weight. This follow-up research suggests that the neutral IAT findings may not mean that Paraguayans haven't internalized weight stigma. Instead, it's possible that they just haven't had anti-fat thoughts for long enough for it to have become a practiced pattern yet.[33]

Back in the Pacific, other ethnographers are starting to paint a similar picture of ambiguity and ambivalence around fat. A three-hour flight to the north of Fiji, in the least traveled part of the Pacific, is the tiny nation of Nauru. Alex used to travel through Nauru regularly. It is a singular and isolated place, where energetic British guano mining operations removed the topsoil and with it the traditional crops. Almost all foodstuffs are now imported. A single, circular road around the island and high levels of car ownership mean that people get little exercise. Figuring out ways to be physically active in the equatorial heat, with a lack of places to go, is a challenge. For these reasons, Nauru has long been labeled as "the fattest country on Earth." It's a distressing claim to fame for Nauruans who know that the world has declared them outstandingly unhealthy and defined them nationally by their high obesity rates. In response, Nauru has stopped reporting its obesity rates to the World Health Organization and it no longer appears on the annual list.

Australian anthropologist Amy McLennan recently spent a year talking to Nauruans about bodies, fat, and life there. McLennan explains how time spent each day socializing ("yarning") with others is seen as key to being well and happy. The obligation to spend time yarning also means that Nauruans feel they don't have time to fit in other things like exercising, even if they believe they *should*. In this context, people feel that if others see them spending time on activities to control their weight, they may view this as a lack of comparable and expected effort to connect with and support others.[34] Consequently, the Nauruan moral meanings of fat bodies are a complex mix of positive (being a good friend) and negative (being unhealthy) at the same time.

In her recent study of the meanings of food in Samoa, our collaborator, cultural anthropologist Jessica Hardin, has also shown how people simultaneously apply multiple, conflicted meanings to large bodies.[35] Highly religious, Samoans see piety, power, and godliness in large bodies. Churches validate largeness as fitting in, part of community feasting, and other important social activities. However, antiobesity and diabetes public health campaigns, which have existed for decades in Samoa, have also generated and made people adopt bad ("unhealthy") messages around fat. Weight-related teasing and fat jokes are common. Hardin has explained that the presence of these competing cultural models, saying that fat is both bad and good, means the teasing and jokes around weight seem to hurt people far less.

While these forms of body ambiguity may make fat less emotionally taxing, it doesn't mean they don't ultimately damage people's health. Psychological anthropologist Anne Becker has been doing ethnographic work on body image in neighboring Fiji since the 1980s.[36] As it has in all central Pacific nations, eating in Fiji remains fully intertwined in the social fabric. Care of others is communicated by giving people plenty of food, and love means encouraging consumption. We bring Arizona State University global health undergraduate students to Fiji for a village stay each year, just down the road from where Becker does her research. Eating is always a major and fabulous part of the stay. As village guests, we are welcomed with feasts of fish, pork, chicken, taro roots and leaves, breadfruit, rice, and bread. Eating goes on for hours and we are constantly encouraged to eat as much as we can.

Becker's work has explained how the large body of a well-fed Fijian (and visitor) demonstrates the caring and the support of family and friends. It expresses love. A skinny body screams neglect and brings shame to the family. But more recently, with a new idolization of slimness gaining traction, young Fijians have been struggling to build bodies that are slim and muscular at the same time. By being slim and muscular, you can communicate the love of family and village (being fed), while also confirming you are modern and worldly (being slim). Young girls are now using both purgatives and appetite stimulants in a complex plan designed to create a body neither too fat nor too slim. The result is an epidemic of eating disorders in Fiji, a factor that is well-established as an easy trigger for depression.

Surely not Everyone?

But surely not *everyone, everywhere* is buying into the belief that fat is always bad? One place we initially guessed that we might find people immune to fat stigma—even as body weight, incomes, and education go up—are places where women's bodies are never on public display. What about places like the United Arab Emirates (UAE), where there are strict dress codes and serious penalties for showing uncovered images of women, and where two-thirds of adults are now overweight? Our collaborator, cultural anthropologist Sarah Trainer, has conducted hundreds of hours of participant observation in the UAE with women university students. She hung out on campus, at coffee shops, and in homes. All the women she interviewed greatly respected local tradition and law. They dressed in the *abaya* (overgarment) and *shayla* (head covering or veil). They never went anywhere without family permission. They also knew well that their families didn't want them to be too skinny. Amani, for example, explained, "A girl who 'filled out her skin' . . . showed her family had enough to feed her well . . . my grandmother always tries to feed me."[37]

And yet, Trainer also found these young women spent extraordinary and extreme worry and effort on avoiding *any* appearance of fat. They embraced extreme dieting and squeezed into elastic girdles (aka *Spanx*). They saw fat as unhealthy and were well-aware of the global media coverage of rising obesity and the thin-idealism of the fashion world. The magazines they read were filled with pictures of scantily clad pop and social media stars. Foreign movies and soap operas depicted thin, glamorous women in revealing and expensive dresses. They were bombarded with advertising for skin care, fashion, and diet products. Fat for them was intolerable. It had become symbolic of being lazy and backward, out-of-date and ignorant of the ways of the modern world. It also sparked vicious teasing by other girls. For young women in the UAE, fat had to be avoided at all costs.

So, we then tried a different tack. We wondered about places where food shortages are common. Wouldn't constant worry about getting enough to eat make fat seem like a good thing? Our collaborator cultural anthropologist Jonathan Maupin interviewed hundreds of adults and children in the relatively small, rural town of Acatenango in the Guatemalan highlands in 2013 to help us figure this out (figure 4.3).[38] Guatemala has one of the highest rates in the world of the so-called "dual burden" of over- and under-malnutrition. Some families within communities are struggling with food insecurity and others aren't. Bodies in Acatenango range from extremely thin to very fat.[39]

Maupin began visiting Acatenango as a child, when his grandfather started the regional medical clinic. He has personally witnessed decades of hunger in the town. More recently, he has also watched the rise in obesity and an increase in chronic diseases like diabetes that are now straining the clinic. He asked adults in Acatenango to list

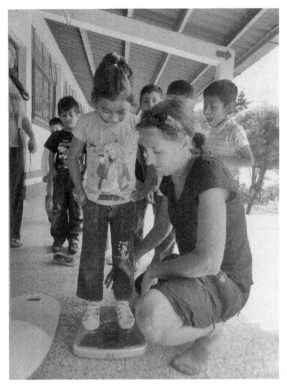

Figure 4.3.   An ASU global health student measuring children's weights at the school in Acatenango, Guatemala, 2013. Photo by J. Maupin

adjectives they knew to describe bodies, both good and bad. Common answers were "intelligent," "strong," "ugly," and "lazy." He then worked with the school to interview and weigh most of the children in the town. Each schoolchild was given drawings of differently sized bodies and asked to match them with a preselected list of these adjectives.

Maupin found that the children of Acatenango had few kind words to say about larger bodies.[40] They called them "ugly" and "lazy." Overweight children in the village also told Maupin stories of being teased because of their weight. He saw bullying firsthand during visits to the school. Given Acatenango is rural and poor and in the global south, this finding of widespread weight cruelty was unanticipated and new. But we also found that the food insecure students attached a lot of negative words to thin bodies too, and thin teasing was also quite common. It turns out that, for young people in Acatenango, you shouldn't be fat—but you shouldn't be too thin either.[41]

We have worked with Maupin more recently to analyze national data for a larger sample of 12,074 Guatemalan women. The goal was to see if evidence of damaging weight stigma extends beyond Acatenango. We detected amazingly high levels of weight teasing and mistreatment across all of Guatemala.[42] Importantly, this unwanted body teasing is extremely distressing. Those women reporting weight-related teasing were 2.1 times more likely to report mild distress and 3.7 times more likely to report moderate-to-severe symptoms of anxiety/depression. Importantly, risk of body teasing was highest in women who were already vulnerable in other ways—those who are younger, poorer, and less food secure. In the analysis, we found that the emotional impact of weight-related teasing on mental health was similar to living through civil war, domestic abuse, and hunger. For Guatemalans at least, anti-fat ideas are being deeply internalized as self-stigma[43] and this is driving a wave of subclinical depression. We suspect this is just one glimpse of a much larger, powerful, depressing, and damaging wave of self-doubt that now spans the globe— one that is developing and spreading without much notice.

The Bottom Line

Socially acceptable, discriminatory, anti-fat attitudes are deepening and spreading. Fat stigma is now a global problem. Its rapid and recent rise shows how new stigmas can emerge almost invisibly but powerfully. In places where large bodies were historically highly valued, this doesn't seem to be protective. Instead, we see the emergence of dual demands where people are trying to avoid being too fat and too thin at the same time. This seems to be driving new epidemics of disordered eating and depression.

5

The Tyranny of Weight Judgment

The powerful and socially tolerated stigma of extreme weight is embedded in a set of widely accepted and deeply ingrained beliefs. We just *know* them to be true, regardless of the actual scientific evidence. Together, these shape our globalizing views of what fat people *are* and what their weight really *means*. Let's explore this by separating the cultural facts from the medical ones.

Cultural Belief 1: You Control Your Weight! Weight Loss Is Easy!

There is clear and consistent scientific evidence that the powerful predictors of obesity in places like the United States include advancing age, poverty, policies (such as commuter transportation, medical care coverage), and spatial factors (such as neighborhood disamenities) that more greatly affect groups that are marginalized or disadvantaged to begin with (such as minorities).[1] Yet, most people believe that adults with extreme weights are fully at fault for their predicament.[2] As an example, take the readers' online comments in response to another, more recent article covering our work in the *New York Times*. The article discussed the fat shaming of a former Miss Universe by then-presidential candidate Donald Trump. One reader had this to say,

The difference between being fat and being black, disabled, or female is that all the latter traits are not under your control. You cannot be blamed for being born with a particular skin color, gender or disability. But your weight IS under your control. Being fat is the result of eating too much for your metabolism and lifestyle. No amount of empty verbiage will change this simple fact. People have predispositions toward a particular body type but nobody is fated to weigh 300 pounds if they don't consume more calories than they expend in their daily activities. Being fat is about the failure of the will to control your food intake. So no, I don't feel guilty when a fat woman in the clothing store winces when I ask for a size 4 dress when she cannot get into a 14. And what am I supposed to do? Gain weight to make fat people feel better?

And many people maintain the problem is laziness and lack of effort:

The vast majority of people do have a choice. People lose weight all the time. There's an entire TV industry that documents morbidly obese people losing weight (Heavy, the Biggest Loser) . . . People are deluding themselves to believe that it can't be done. Obviously, it can.

The "fatties" are also blamed for everything from uncomfortable public transportation to sky-high health costs, to unreasonable carbon footprints, and endangering unborn babies' lives. As a result, many, such as this reader, reason that they get what they deserve for their "poor choices"—utter social rejection.

Everybody has known for at least the last 10 years that a regular diet of fast food and sodas is bad for you just like smoking yet people CHOOSE these poor options at their own expense and others . . . they should not be led to believe it's okay unless they want to live exclusively among those of their ilk.

Ln, New York, April 1, 2011

A core cultural idea underpinning these comments is that weight is always an *individual* responsibility. People think your body directly reflects the amount of effort you put in. Thus, they reason, obesity is created by lack of discipline, laziness, and lack of appropriate effort and care. Fat bodies reflect indulgence in key vices, gluttony and sloth. In contrast, attaining and maintaining slimness reflects our goodness. Weight loss can be achieved by practicing proper self-care and the correct amount of discipline. If you have self-control, weight loss is easy.

People around the world vary in how much they blame individuals for weight gain. Germans and Saudis alike are convinced the key drivers of obesity are poor personal diet or exercise *choices*.[3] Iranians blame government policy, school environments, and personal choices acting together.[4] Where to place blame varies not only between countries but also within societies too, such as along lines of class, gender, and body size. Lower-income Brazilians stress the roles of heredity and stress. High-income Brazilians, especially those who aren't obese, place greater blame on poor diet and exercise choices.[5] Perhaps not surprisingly, Brazil's government has focused on strategies that use media programs to "teach" people (especially lower-income groups) how to eat, live, and be healthier through better self-control.

In 2012, we launched a new project in partnership with the Mayo Clinic's bariatric (weight-loss surgery) clinic in Phoenix, Arizona (figure 5.1). We followed and repeatedly interviewed thirty-five women and men as they went through weight-loss surgeries and for two years afterward. At the same time, we also collected survey data with three hundred other patients who had gone through the same surgery within the Mayo Clinic hospital system in the preceding five years.[6] The goal was to understand how people deal with the stigma of extreme weight and how that connects with their efforts to lose it. In the course of that project, our research team learned much from people struggling through myriad, repeated efforts to slim down "by themselves." All of the patients in the study were considered "morbidly obese" when they arrived at the bariatric clinic. Many had been technically "obese"—and felt fat—for much of their lives. After years of listening to what patients shared, we now fully understand that people who resort to surgery have years of repeated, humiliating failures to lose weight behind them. People are utterly determined to do whatever is needed to succeed.

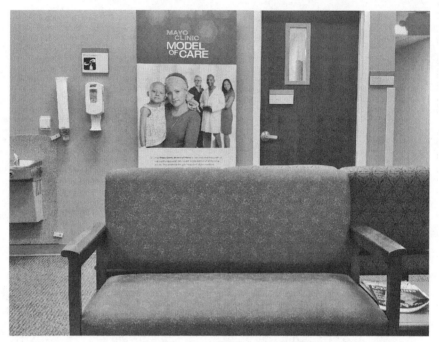

Figure 5.1. Chairs in the general waiting room area at Mayo Clinic in Arizona, designed to fit all sized bodies. Too few medical and other public spaces are designed to allow for larger bodies. Photo by A. Brewis

Sarah Trainer, having finished her long-term fieldwork on women's body issues in the United Arab Emirates, led the data collection in this study, repeatedly interviewing patients before, during, and in the years following their surgeries. Bariatric surgery is a long, detailed, and committed process at the Mayo Clinic. The surgery itself causes your stomach to be shrunk and your intestines rerouted. But, at the Mayo Clinic, healthcare for bariatric patients is much more extensive and holistic. Patients have to go through complex dietary training and practice prior to surgery. After the surgery, they must comply with complicated dietary rules. Recovery itself can be challenging, as the body copes with the surgery and its aftermath. Enormous weight loss is almost guaranteed—at least in first year.

However, with major weight loss comes new challenges, such as uncomfortable, loose skin. Those new dietary rules—which patients have to obey for the rest of their lives—are strict and difficult to follow. If a patient breaks them, they could suffer "dumping," a condition in which food gets painfully pushed into the small intestine without being digested. People told us it feels like being stabbed by sharp knives or swallowing razor blades. In other words, even weight-loss surgery, considered by many to be the "easy way out" of obesity, requires an extraordinary amount of work, effort, and commitment.

In fact, if we use number of days dieting as the metric, the people who put the *most effort* into weight loss are actually those who are classified as morbidly obese. As one especially empathetic endocrinologist colleague at the Mayo Clinic said to us, "What is more heroic than trying something really hard again and again even though you know it is likely to fail?" If we wanted to actually support people's weight-loss efforts, viewing the morbidly obese as heroes—people who are fighting against heredity, environmental constraints, and changing food environments—would be a more helpful cultural maxim. But it isn't the one that dominates. Instead, most people see fat and think "failure."

Even when someone manages to lose the weight, the stigma often persists. And this persistent stigma seems to make maintaining weight loss harder. For example, in the surveys of those three hundred post-bariatric patients, we found that those who had the highest levels of stigma were likely to have more difficulty following the recommended postsurgical diet and exercise regimes. They had more significantly disordered eating habits, ate more calories and items considered less healthy (like ice cream and alcohol), and were less willing to exercise in public places (like jogging outdoors, lifting weights at the gym, or visiting the local swimming pool). The effect was unrelated to how much weight people started with or had lost, rather it was all about how much stigma they had internalized.

What we discovered from the detailed, patient interviews was that those they interacted with at work or elsewhere in their everyday worlds would suggest that weight loss only "counts" as a personal success if it also proves you have managed the requisite self-discipline. Thus weight-loss surgery or new-line pharmaceuticals that promote major weight loss are widely viewed as "cheating." Accordingly, many bariatric patients are very selective about who they tell about their surgeries and were worried others would judge them even as they lost weight simply on the basis of having had the surgery. This is why they are at pains to point out how much work they had to do to lose the weight before and after surgery.[7] It is really hurtful to not get moral credit when you do what society told you was required. One bariatric patient, Sally, told Trainer, "I had one person say to me, 'Well, you did it the easy way' . . . He will never say that again. I lashed out at him. He got it full force and he will never say that again. I mean, if you think having surgery and going through what I went through is easy, I said, 'You've got a lot to learn.'"[8]

The basic idea that you control your own weight and that weight loss is merely a matter of self-control is reflected in most medical and public health approaches to obesity. When you talk to a doctor, the advice they give is focused on the effort you should be making: exercise more and eat less to meet the requisite body mass index (BMI) goals.[9] In public health, this is termed the "behavior-change" approach. It tries to change people's attitudes and, thereby, adjust their eating and exercise "choices." Motivating behavior change is often done via health communication, whether through a doctor's advice, through posters and television spots, or through other forms of social influence. As with the handwashing example in part I, an assumption of the behavior-change model is that we must eliminate ignorance.

And yet, despite much public education, there is really no good example of any country managing to reverse the obesity epidemic to date. This failure isn't due to flat-out ignorance, because whenever we survey people—anywhere in the world—everyone already *knows* the eat less/exercise more mantra. Nor is it caused by a lack of widespread personal effort. People at high body weights actually diet *more* often than the general population.

The failure to stop the obesity epidemic is instead related to the underestimation of the real and sustained efforts that people with the largest bodies invest in trying to lose weight. When people are handed the personal responsibility of trying to lose weight, most fail.[10]

The current estimates suggest one in twenty people that lose weight manage to keep it off long-term. The behavior-change model is so fully ingrained in how we approach obesity that we seem to ignore the growing scientific evidence that it is a failing strategy, and that there is a better one.

Alex wrote a book about obesity in 2011 that presents the argument that the most effective way to curb obesity is through hard-to-make structural changes.[11] Things like making cities more walkable, shaping classrooms to be activity-focused, providing healthier food options, and addressing poverty are the difficult yet ultimately successful changes that will decrease obesity. Moreover, underpinning these efforts is a very different cultural belief: Removing excess weight is a shared responsibility that will require sustained, collective effort. To fix obesity no one should ever struggle alone, and yet, that is all people seem to be doing.

Cultural Belief 2: Fat Is Dangerous!

Another highly influential cultural belief that defies medical fact is that the obese body is *always* unhealthy. The fat body is thus seen as a dangerous body—one that is killing itself. In addition, it is seen to be damaging the rest of us by extension. There is no doubt that very high levels of obesity are associated with a long list of medical conditions that lead to serious illness and disability, such as diabetes, arthritis, sleep apnea, high blood pressure, high cholesterol, and soft tissue infections. But it isn't always or inevitable that people with high levels of body fat are unhealthy. There is growing understanding of "metabolically healthy obesity." This is the idea that you can be overweight but still have excellent physiological markers of health. Certainly, a substantial subpopulation of obese people—especially those who exercise regularly—are free of any weight-related diseases. In the same manner, people who are so-called "normal" weight—especially those not getting regular exercise or with very poor diets—can have metabolic profiles (high blood sugar, high cholesterol, high blood pressure) that look like ones we associate with obesity. In other words, we have culturally conflated the correct association between poor diet and little exercise and physical danger with the incorrect assumption that "fat" equals unhealthy.

Moreover, these days we think of obesity as a *disease*, which is a pretty arbitrary call. The American Medical Association (AMA) only declared it a disease in 2014 after long-term discussion about whether obesity *in itself* (i.e., without other associated medical conditions) is a deviation from a healthy bodily state. This suggests that the AMA recognizes that it is at least debatable whether obesity is itself a disease, rather than just signifying the likelihood of other diseases.[12] In fact, their own Council on Science and Public Health argued that, "Given the existing limitations of B.M.I. to diagnose obesity in clinical practice, it is unclear that recognizing obesity as a disease, as opposed to a 'condition' or 'disorder,' will result in improved health outcomes."

Cultural Belief 3: The Helping Professions Help

There are so many people whose job is to help us lose weight. But primary care physicians, nutritionists, and personal trainers are like everyone else: They, too, are shaped by these cultural ideas and endorse weight stigma, either consciously or unconsciously. UCLA psychologist Janet Tomiyama has been studying weight stigma for over a decade. She recently designed a fascinating study to use IAT to measure the internalized weight stigma of attendees at a major scientific and medical international conference on obesity called *Obesity-Week*. By comparing her results to similar IAT tests done with the same conference attendees a decade earlier, she found that negative judgment of fat people had actually increased. People's stigmatizing reaction times had become faster.[13] In other words, the very people whose job is to help others lose weight have been becoming more prejudiced against them.

Many studies have shown that anti-fat attitudes are harbored at the very core of medicine. Larger medical students report high levels of derogatory humor or derogatory comments about their weight from their peers and instructors. Trainee nurses and doctors avoid obesity-related specialties because they are viewed as a less rewarding or rewarded career path.[14]

Patients who don't lose weight are viewed as difficult and hard to treat, as noncompliant "failures." Yet, primary care physicians spend less time consulting with obese patients than non-obese patients. They also expend less effort in establishing emotional rapport, such as being empathetic, reassuring, and involving patients in medical decision-making.[15] Many see consults with obese patients simply as a waste of their time. And the heavier the patient, the more they report they didn't enjoy the work or lost their patience.[16] Apparently, doctors also trust their patients less: Those struggling unsuccessfully to lose weight report doctors will imply they are lying when they tell them they have been following the diet or exercise prescriptions, but they don't lose weight.

Given the cultural myth that obesity is always extremely unhealthy, clinicians often focus on an obese patient's weight during consultations even if the patient is there for entirely unrelated reasons. Similarly, slimmer people with unhealthy metabolic profiles are often not counseled to make lifestyle changes, because their doctors assume they are healthy. As one of our bariatric study participants put it, "You know, you go in there, 'I got a headache.' [The doctor says] 'It's because you're fat.' 'My toes hurt.' 'It's because you're fat.'"

The website First Do No Harm[17] is replete with people's stories of doctors refusing to diagnose and treat serious illnesses because they remain convinced that any health problem in someone classified as obese *must* stem from their weight. Take Katie, for example, whose walking pneumonia was missed because the doctor was convinced she had obesity-triggered sleep apnea. Or Rachel, who was congratulated for losing so much weight, which turned out to be the result of debilitating Crohn's disease. Or Erica, who was struck by a drunk driver and seriously injured, but the ER doctor decided he couldn't set her broken arm because of her size.

Even when doctors try their best, the gowns, chairs, and medical equipment don't fit extremely obese people. As one patient explained,

"A doctor's surgery is not, and has never been, a safe place . . . The AMA's decision to further medicalize my body and refer to it as diseased—a body that I love, a body that is carrying me around with no health problems, is just another reason for me to fear the medical establishment that wants to hurt me and have me thank them for it."[18]

Unsurprisingly, many people struggling with their weight feel mistreated. They forego any noncritical visits such as annual checkups or cancer screenings.[19] They "doctor shop," moving from practice to practice to find someone they feel comfortable with. Accordingly, they end up with worse continuity of care,[20] or they refuse to engage with the unwelcoming medical system at all. All of this means that, while the anti-fat attitudes that seep into patient care are painful emotionally, they also have wider, unwanted, public health impacts such as lower rates of referral and diagnosis of other deadly conditions like cancer.

Fat activists, those pushing for better treatment of large people, have provided clear guidelines for how clinicians can help improve the patient experience. These include understanding the upstream and complex causes of obesity, the psychological and emotional burdens of weight and weight stigma, and being willing to stick with patients over the long term.[21] While this doesn't seem like a lot, the reality for most morbidly obese patients is that they find it difficult to forge empathetic, long-term relationships with clinicians. Emerging efforts to include "structural competence" training for medical school students should help, because it is designed to help future clinicians to better recognize the broader social and political forces that shape who gets sickest and why.

Cultural Belief 4: Shame Spurs Weight Loss!

There's one more key prevailing cultural belief that is common in both the media and medicine: Fat stigma *helps* motivate people to lose weight. As the United Kingdom's public health minister told the BBC, doctors *should* call patients "fat" because it will motivate people to lose weight and to take more personal responsibility. Again, this is exemplified in our *New York Times* reader comments, one of whom said, "Let's have more stigma against fat people. Not less. More stigma would help fat people do what they can't do on their own. Eat less." But the scientific evidence does not support this. Actually, weight stigma actively *undermines* the possibility of weight loss and ultimately leads to longer-term weight gain. For this reason, we should be concerned that chronic experiences of weight stigma are a largely unrecognized and powerful driver of the obesity epidemic.

So how does this extremely ironic process work? There are several different mechanisms that contribute.[22] One factor is that fat stigma makes people not want to go out in public to exercise. If you feel others are judging you, you are less likely to want to jog in a park, swim in a public pool, or join a sports team. Our studies with bariatric surgery patients reinforced this, even when patients were losing substantial weight after their surgeries. Many had chronically encountered fat stigma in everyday life for so long that they personally endorsed it. This *internalized* stigma—rather than actual experiences when they were out exercising—made them hesitant to be physically active.

We have observed other ways that negative feedback loops between weight stigma and obesity function among undergraduates on the ASU campus, right outside our office windows. We often pilot the tools we design for our international, weight stigma research on campus with students, since they come from 120 countries. Using ASU as our test bed has also yielded a lot of information about weight stigma on our own campus. To begin, we conducted surveys of weight stigma and its effects on students' health-relevant behaviors using a geographically randomized sample of 445 students in 2013.[23] More recently, in 2015 and 2016, we worked with our nutritionist colleague, Meg Breuning, who led a systematic effort to collect data on diet, exercise, weight stigma, and friendship in 1,443 freshmen students living in the Arizona State University residence halls during their first year.[24]

Through these various studies, we've found that ASU is a typical university in three ways: A lot of students worry about weight, many students have high weights, and students on average gain a significant amount of weight during the years they are in college. About 10 percent have a BMI greater than thirty, meaning about 8,500 of our students are clinically defined as "obese."

In addition, from interviewing and measuring thousands of students over the last five years, we can say with some certainty that anti-fat thinking is the norm on campus.[25] Our students exhibit extremely high levels of implicit weight stigma (i.e., what they are *thinking*), and reasonably high levels of explicit weight stigma (i.e., what they are *saying*), compared to other US and international populations.[26]

Our studies on our own Arizona State University campus also show that students with high body weights really *feel* this judgment. Some 15 percent of the students surveyed felt so ashamed of their bodies that they actively avoided public events and making friends as a means to cope, and this wasn't just the students with the largest bodies saying this. But those students that are technically "obese" are those that more often tell us in one-on-one interviews that campus is often a particularly unwelcoming and unfriendly place for them. Large bodies can't fit them into lecture hall seating and getting through campus parking lots is a struggle. There is plenty of direct, cruel discrimination on display, too, once you start to pay attention. For example, "No Fat Chicks" bumper stickers are displayed with pride. In our interviews, we discovered the place on campus where people felt the most weight stigma was ironically the recreation center. The huge mirrors in the workout rooms made people feel especially uncomfortable. As a result, many larger students said they avoided the gym altogether. The interview data also showed that feeling fat stigma breeds exercise avoidance. Breuning's more detailed tracking of students' exercise for an entire year also showed the same thing: Those who felt more stigmatized were less likely to want to exercise, including those who weren't even overweight. And they were more likely to be depressed.

In addition, exposure to weight stigma, such as through teasing or even just viewing slim-centric media images, seems to make it harder for people to control their eating, as we noted above in our findings from the Mayo Clinic study. It particularly triggers comfort eating, bingeing, and yo-yo dieting. People who are already overweight seem most susceptible.[27] For example, bariatric patients with greater levels of internalized stigma had the hardest time following the complex, post-bariatric dietary guidelines.[28] All these types of "disordered" eating and exercise avoidance can reset body metabolism and change appetite cues. As such, they help to promote weight gain over the longer-term, reinforcing the negative feedback loop.[29]

Just feeling stigmatized in itself can trigger weight-inducing stress responses within the body. In one illuminating study, Janet Tomiyama's team borrowed an idea from "top model" Tyra Banks's infamous fat suit experiment (figure 5.2).[30] They asked half of their participants to don a regular shirt and pants. They had the other half put on a shirt and pants that looked the same but were much larger, with a fat suit underneath. The participants walked around in public on a predetermined route. When they got back to the lab, the fat-suited participants reported feeling more anger, anxiety, sadness, hurt, and rejection. They also ate more of the candy and drank more of the soda that Tomiyama's lab team gave them. And, importantly, their cortisol levels shot up as well. Cortisol is one of the main reactive stress hormones in our endocrine system. For those already overweight, chronic activation of cortisol leads to additional weight gain over time.[31]

The physiological stress from weight stigma not only affects those who are overweight, but also "normal"-sized people. In another experiment, Tomiyama's team recruited UCLA students to participate in a "shopping" experiment. Once in the study, half of the students were told they couldn't continue because their size and shape were wrong for trying on "fashionable clothing." Regardless of their weight, those who were told that they weren't the right size for the study had significant rises in cortisol compared to others. Considering the constant stigma and discrimination experienced by people with large bodies,[32] it is easy to see how increased cortisol from such constant rejection could drive up weight over time. One study found larger women reported an average of twenty-two stigmatizing events in just one week of tracking, including nasty comments and public staring.[33]

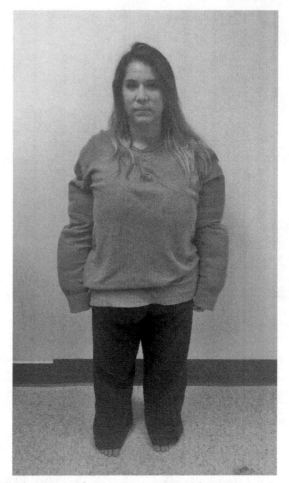

Figure 5.2. The "fat suit" used for Janet Tomiyama's weight stigma experiments at UCLA. Photo courtesy of J. Tomiyama

Feeling weight stigma also, unsurprisingly, leads to depression, and research shows that depression, and the pills used to treat it, in turn, spur yet more weight gain.[34] In the last several years, we have analyzed large, longitudinal data sets from across the globe to see if the pattern is persistent. We have found that results are always much the same, whether for new mothers in Norway or middle-aged men in Korea. The more people worry about being overweight, the more depressed they become over time and the more weight they gain.

Whenever weight stigma triggers strong, negative, internalized responses it has the potential to make weight gain more likely and harder to reverse. Moreover, because exposure to stigma and discrimination only magnifies as people get fatter,[35] it is a slippery downhill slide to full-on misery.

Shoot the Messenger

Media, public health and medical messaging around the "obesity epidemic" all constantly reinforce the idea that excess fat is dangerous, deadly, and against the public interest.[36] Headlines we've seen include the colorful "Aporkerlypse now" (*The Sun*); "Obesity as Dangerous as Terror Threat" (*The Times*); and "Big Mums Risk Babies' Health" (*New Zealand Herald*).[37] This type of dramatic media coverage that highlights the perils of obesity has been escalating for years.[38]

Media coverage of obesity matters because it shapes and reflects our ideas about both causation and blame. From news reporting of public health and medical findings, we learn much of what we know about why people gain weight, and how it and they should be treated. Generally, the media focus heavily on poor lifestyle decisions (eating too much, exercising too little) as the explanation for *why* people are fat.[39] There is less examination of structural reasons for growing obesity rates, such as inadequate transportation systems that give people little choice but to drive to work. The media gives short shrift to schools' trend to cut recess time to save money, which forces schoolchildren to spend more of their day sitting. We don't often hear stories about why high-carb, processed foods are cheaper and more accessible, making them a rational choice for people living in poverty.

Individual blame remains a constant theme. Not surprisingly, many legislators—who read the news but not the scientific studies being cited—assume that increased individual levels of physical activity will reduce obesity. However, there is absolutely no scientific evidence of this, even if it does improve health.[40]

The reporting of obesity as an *epidemic*[41] is based on a popularized version of the messages coming from medicine and public health about the rising chronic disease risks associated with it. Such stories seem to suggest at some level that obesity (or rather obese people) damage society. When we were in Ireland in 2014, a major government investment was underway to enhance people's physical activity by encouraging sports and other social exercise. The prominent public face of obesity prevention efforts was endocrinologist Donal O'Shea, brother of Irish rugby star Conor O'Shea. He was constantly cited in the media, saying things such as, "But if we don't address the obesity epidemic, we're just going to continue feeding cancer into waiting lists, feeding diabetes into waiting lists."[42] He provided fodder for headlines like "Ireland's obesity problem will be worse than cholera or Aids for our health service, Professor warns."[43]

The images of obese people that accompany such media reporting also reinforce stigma. One analysis of five major media sources showed that almost three-quarters of all images of overweight or obese people

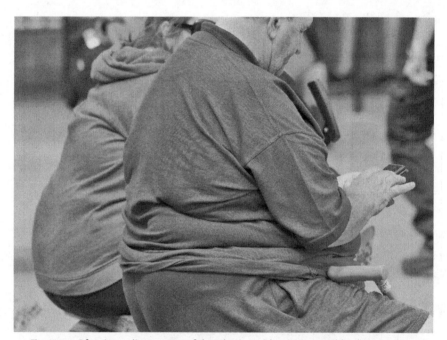

Figure 5.3. Often in media coverage of the "obesity epidemic," images like this one are cropped to focus on a headless torso eating unhealthy foods, giving the impression that the person is defined by their size. © Shutterstock

were fundamentally dehumanizing (figure 5.3). Examples include shots of headless bodies and faces depicted as places to shove cheeseburgers.

Of course, there are differences around the world in exactly how the blame for obesity is apportioned. In Ireland, failure to get involved in popular social sports like rugby pops up commonly. In Australia, mothers tend to get more than a fair dose of blame in the media. A recent headline there read, "Family Meals Cut Teenage Fatness," and another reporter boldly claimed, "The research suggests women who are overweight before they fall pregnant, and during it, may be condemning their children to a life of overeating and obesity."[44]

The media also reports on people who defy or overcome weight prejudice and stigma, but the way they are portrayed still reinforces the notion that being fat is "not normal." Overweight dancers, for example, are invariably described as "brave" and "challenging discrimination." For example, 15-year-old ballerina Lizzy Howell "Challenges Body Stereotypes,"[45] Whitney Thor is reported to dance as a form of plus-size "activism,"[46] and the Cuban dance troupe *Danza Voluminosa* ("Voluminous Dance") are called "courageous" to dance while fat.[47]

Beyond the news, television shows contribute to reinforcing and growing stigma too. Overweight people are rarely portrayed as the love interest. Fashionable people are skinny. Insulting "fattertainment" is everywhere. These reality shows convey a fictional, scientific narrative about how everyone can and must manage their weight.[48] The format on one British show, *You Are What You Eat*, consists of shaming the obese participant by laying out an array of all the (unhealthy) foods they eat in a typical week. This is followed by a truly humiliating analysis of their feces so the host (a nutritionist) can prove if they are being dishonest about their "deadly" dietary choices.

The extremely popular show *The Biggest Loser* is one of the most watched—and hence influential—shows about losing weight. The format encourages, cajoles, and shames obese contestants into losing colossal amounts of weight through diet and exercise over a twelve-week season.[49] It reinforces the idea that one cannot be happy or successful and large at the same time. We certainly share the concerns of others that the show isn't helping people create better lives; it cheapens the struggle to lose weight and seems to drive the audience to have *less* empathy for those who are overweight.[50]

By making extreme weight loss look quick and easy, shows like *The Biggest Loser* reinforce that anyone who remains fat is just being lazy. In one study, undergraduates who reported watching more of these shows were more likely to believe that body weight is under personal control and obesity is due to personal responsibility.[51] All this "fat porn" is really not helping anyone—except perhaps those who make a living from television ratings. And it's going international too. During Amber's last fieldwork trip to Paraguay, people were buzzing about the latest episode of *Cuestión de Peso* ("Weighty Matters"), an Argentine version of *The Biggest Loser*. This is after *The Biggest Loser* has apparently gone into hiatus in the United States in the midst of growing questions around both the medical mistreatment and the massive weight regain of contestants.[52]

The Inescapability of Fat Stigma

I've been big all my life . . . I guess you would call it super obese, but I hate those words . . . As a wife, it makes you unsure about yourself and whether your spouse is truly attracted to you. My husband reassures me all the time that I am beautiful, but the problem lies in myself that I don't believe that I am . . . There are times, I just don't want to leave the house or my room even. I don't want to go anywhere or see anyone. I joke that I wish I could call in 'fat' like some people call in 'sick.' You can't escape it. I was at Disneyland for my son's Make-a-Wish trip and got stuck in the turnstiles. I feel ashamed of myself because I can't get up the energy to care what awful shape I have let my body and health get to . . . If only I could lose the weight and become the person I want to be. Honestly, at this point I don't think it's ever going to happen. I'm just not strong enough.

Coleen, Scottsdale, Arizona, United States, 2012

The misery of the fat stigma portrayed in media and health messages is very intensely felt by people with large bodies. One of the main reasons is that the messages are so pervasive and inescapable. You can't just unplug and be safe. They remind you that you should be skinny, that you don't fit in the physical world. Every movement in public spaces can remind you of how you are not "normal." You can't buy your "abnormal"-sized clothes in regular stores. Just visiting a restaurant can be a nightmare. The booths don't fit, and worse, people judge every bite you eat. If you eat pie, expect sideways looks and sneers. Other than complete social withdrawal, there are few ways to avoid the constant cruelty.

This explicit stigma cannot be easily managed in public settings because—unlike many other types of stigmatized conditions—there is no way for people to hide their weight when out in the world. With HIV or herpes, you might decide not to share your diagnosis with everyone you meet. But very large bodies cannot be hidden or denied, so "passing" as skinny in public is just not an option. Furthermore, for many stigmas—like physical disabilities or a cancer diagnosis—family and friends can provide a space of refuge, of acceptance and relief. This is often not the case with weight stigma, for which family and friends can be the cruelest. Those closest to you may feel it is okay to note that you shouldn't be eating dessert, even if everyone else is. They find it within reason to tell you they are embarrassed to be seen in public with you. They are happy to provide unsolicited, soul-crushing weight loss and exercise advice or giggle when you struggle to fit in a seatbelt.

This is not to say that people don't deploy a wide array of strategies to cope with this hurtful, everyday treatment. They do. People may do things like staying at home and avoiding social contact, breaking with family, working to become indifferent, or stepping out as a proud fat activist. At the same time, though, one of the real challenges of weight is that it can't be hidden: In regular social interactions, bodies are omni-visible.

A couple of years ago, we began to wonder if new, online environments might be a safer space for people struggling with weight. We thought maybe they could help people try to lose weight without having to worry about what observers thought. We started by analyzing blogs, since online bloggers, theoretically, have a great deal of control over how they present their bodies and stories to an audience. Our hope was that weight-loss bloggers, including those with higher initial body weights, would feel empowered by their weight-loss efforts, regardless of whether they lost weight or not. During 2014–2015, we tracked the date-stamped entries of 234 active bloggers based in the United States. We then analyzed their writing for themes such as weight-loss success, weight-loss failure, and body acceptance.[53] Unfortunately, these results show that virtual worlds are often just as miserable for people struggling with their weight. The texts were riddled with laments over the authors' failure to lose weight. Bloggers confessed their lack of discipline, failure at self-control, and failure to eat or exercise as they believed they "should." Even worse, the few bloggers that embraced fat-positive views and encouraged self-acceptance became targeted by vicious trolling. Weight stigma appears to be inescapable, even when the body is invisible.

The Beneficiaries

When we see stigmatizing cultural ideas that persist despite so much obvious pain and suffering, we always ask: *who benefits*? For example, why would it be important for members of the American Medical Association that obesity is presented as a dangerous disease? One obvious answer is that medical insurance is more likely to cover the cost of weight-loss treatment. Bariatric surgery is currently one of the highest profit-margin medical procedures on offer in the United States.

The focus on obesity as a disease with detrimental medical effects also allows our government legislators, educators, corporations, and city planners to imagine that the solutions to obesity will be found in medical or pharmaceutical treatments. A recent study in Canada,[54] for example, identified near universal support among policy makers for individual-focused policies designed to help people eat less and exercise more. Just like the Community-Led Total Sanitation efforts we explored in part I, responsibility for and the cost of these policies is borne by the consumer (or, in the case of obesity, their insurance company). Consequently, there is less pressure for legislators to address obesity by implementing thoughtful solutions that scientific evidence suggests will be both better and fairer. They are free from pursuing efforts that take time and money, like walkable cities, correcting unhealthy physical workspaces, retooling school curricula, or providing antidiscrimination protections.

A major proliferator of the idea that weight loss is *easy* is the multibillion-dollar diet industry. In the United States alone, some $60 billion is spent annually on people trying to lose weight. Advertising hawks this idea that weight loss is possible for everyone—with just the right product or service. All you need is a master cleanse that will eradicate all carbs and proteins from your diet; a specially designed exercise tool that targets weight loss on the inner thigh; or small, frozen, prepackaged, "healthy" meals that might be low in calories but are extremely high in sodium. All these types of products benefit greatly from the repeated, failed efforts that so many of us go through to lose weight. Unfortunately, their only real goal is profit. Think about it: If people didn't *believe* weight loss could be easily achieved, and it was their job to achieve it—if, instead, they followed the statistics rather than the hype—then weight-loss product sales would plummet.

"Big snack" and "big soda" greatly benefit from the "weight loss is easy" belief, too. As codirector of the Mayo Clinic–ASU "Obesity Solutions" initiative, Alex was once invited to visit with the head of research and development at Kraft, a huge multinational snack company. She was naively expecting the first question to be, "How do we make our products better to help people lose weight or be healthy?" But instead it was, "What can we do to get people to buy more of our products?" This should give everyone pause: No company has been pushing the idea of individual exercise as key to a healthy weight more than Coca-Cola. They (and probably Pepsi, too) have had arguably suspicious relationships with health-promoting charities. For example, Save the

Children, which had promoted soda taxes to improve childhood health, shifted their message following a $5 million donation. Coca-Cola were caught covertly sponsoring a "Global Energy Balance Network" through the University of Colorado School of Medicine, which seriously downplayed the role of diet in weight gain. By these and many other means, multinationals are "lean-washing" their products.[55] If people think that their weight is their own fault, the corporations won't get sued or taxed, and customer boycotts won't damage their profits.

Unfortunately, such tactics damage the most vulnerable fat people the most. Recent research in the United States suggests that the emotional impacts of weight stigma most affect those with less social, economic, or political power. Lower-income women are now showing the greatest emotional and psychological toll.[56]

The Bottom Line

The stigmatizing messages about obesity are communicated constantly—in the schoolyard and on social media; through television casting, advertising, and doctors' advice; in the comments of family members, science reporting in the news, public health service announcements, and corporate sponsorships. This new epidemic of stigma is so riveted into the fabric of our daily lives we take it for granted. It is almost invisible. It is causing profound emotional misery, driving active and legal discrimination, and leaving people with extreme weight on the margins of the health system, unheard and mistreated. Fat stigma is also making us fatter, while making it easier for companies to shirk responsibility and governments to avoid more effective reforms to promote healthier communities.

World War O

New stigmas can emerge and spread easily, as our research on global fat stigma shows. Anti-obesity efforts started globalizing at nearly the same time as new anti-fat ideas. This poses an important question: Could anti-obesity efforts in global public health be fueling the fire, by promoting weight stigma as they try to *fight* obesity?

Global public health efforts around obesity are often alarmist, blaming and shaming, or combative and menacing. The World Health Organization declares obesity "one of the greatest public health challenges of the twenty-first century." The Robert Wood Johnson Foundation tells us that excess fat "threatens [our] future." The US Armed Forces have declared weight a national security threat, rendering a third of their potential recruits unfit to fight.[1] Wealthy, industrialized nations—the so-called global north—have been fighting their *war on obesity*[2] for several decades. Middle-income countries are heading into the same emotionally fraught, expensive battle right now. The lower-income countries, who have to deal with obesity's complicated coexistence with undernutrition, see what is coming for them.

Overweight and obesity are certainly now a truly planetary phenomenon. In countries as diverse as the United States, Egypt, Iceland, Mexico, Hungary, and Saudi Arabia, over two-thirds of adults are now classified as overweight or obese.[3] The United States clocks in at nineteenth on the list of "fattest nations,"[4] with obesity at 67% of the adult population. This means the United States is behind six Pacific Island, two Caribbean, and ten Middle Eastern / Gulf countries. The remainder of the top thirty includes a wide array of countries with rapidly growing or recovering economies. Rough estimates suggest at least two billion people are currently affected, and the numbers are growing quickly.

Obesity's recent and rapid rise is partly due to globalization. Since World War II, processes such as economic growth, market integration, trade liberalization, urbanization, mechanization, and computerization have made high-calorie, high-fat foods cheaper and more accessible. This process has also changed the ways we organize our work, transport, and leisure time, mostly toward inactivity. Until recently, most people in the world did active things to feed their families: growing taro, fishing from a canoe, husbanding camels, or pounding millet. Increasingly, we make our living sitting at a desk. It should be no surprise then that we weigh more.

Increasing physical inactivity started earlier and more slowly in high-income countries like the United States, Canada, and the United Kingdom. In these countries, the rise of obesity is now decades old, and adult obesity rates may even now be plateauing. However, "plateau" is a deceptive word when it involves one-third of adults technically overweight and one-third technically obese. Moreover, child obesity rates continue to rise pretty much everywhere.

In the rest of the world—places like China, South Africa, India, and Brazil—the process started much later but is progressing much, much faster. This has raised serious concerns in many middle-income nations who face projected rises in direct healthcare costs associated with treating chronic, complex, expensive conditions like diabetes and cardiovascular disease. One recent estimate suggests obesity (as a trigger for chronic disease) currently explains more than 20 percent of global healthcare spending. In addition, the indirect costs of obesity include lost workforce productivity due to absenteeism during hospital stays, illness treatment, and long-term disability. In Mexico, that total is estimated to already absorb 2.5 percent of the country's entire GDP.

Mexico, China, and other middle-income nations have already geared up their anti-obesity efforts within the last decade. And now almost every nation is following suit. Even South Korea, the leanest of all the G20 nations with around 5 percent of adults defined as overweight/obese, has begun educating its public about the dangers of weight. And it isn't just governments pushing anti-obesity agendas. Hospitals, non-governmental organizations (NGOs), and private foundations are all pitching in, too. One recent suggestion that has a familiar ring: graphic images of rotting teeth on the side of soda bottles. Australian public health researchers suggest that these visual health warnings in particular, because they are so immediately "revolting and frightening and shocking," could do a good job of putting people off soda, just as they do tobacco.[5] The battle against excess weight has now morphed into a full-on World War O, using disgust as one of its tools.

Shock and Awe

Despite the energy put into these passionate anti-obesity efforts, they have a rather surprising lack of overall strategy and coordination. For infectious disease, public health efforts are often clear and straightforward, with messages like "vaccinate all children against measles." In contrast, for obesity, every group of actors has their own plan. The reasons for this lack of cohesiveness are the complexity and social-structural nature of the problem; a lack of clear science to clarify best practices; and the lack of examples of effective campaigns that have successfully reversed obesity.

The World Health Organization tried to cut through the chaos with a set of solid guidelines about how to address obesity in their 2004 *Global Strategy on Diet, Physical Activity and Health*—but to little avail.[6] Only a few governments have so far designed a set of policies or strategies that fully adhere to the guidelines. Accordingly, local cultural views and idiosyncratic political agendas about weight—differently defining "what fat is" and "why fat matters"—fill in the gaps. In this way, inherently stigmatizing ideas that blame people for their weight easily seep into interventions.

Some of these ideas are what we might call soft stigma. They aren't overtly blaming or shaming, but they fully embrace the idea of individual responsibility in ways that likely reinforce stigmatizing beliefs. For example, take one of the more comprehensive, coordinated anti-obesity efforts in Northern Europe: Iceland's government, school system, and the private sector came together in a national effort to reverse high levels of obesity. They focused on young children who are often viewed as the easiest target for behavior change.

A wildly popular, English-language children's television show, called *LazyTown*, was designed as the centerpiece of Iceland's anti-obesity efforts. The show depicts a colorful, cartoonish place where the villagers are ignorant about healthy food choices and the benefits of exercise. Now shown in over one hundred countries, the archvillain Robbie Rotten encourages kids to enjoy video games and junk food, while hero Sportacus (played by show creator, gymnast, and national hero Magnús Scheving) shows the junk food addicted, video game obsessed, lazy inhabitants that exercise is fun. The approach is not an overtly stigmatizing or shaming one; none of the children in *Lazy-Town* are overweight. They are just portrayed as needing to be saved from their own ignorance.

In Iceland, *LazyTown* was leveraged into a national campaign. All 4-to-7-year-old children were encouraged to make health contracts with their parents.[7] They earned "energy points" by eating "sport candy" (fruit). The participation rates were amazing, with claims that almost 100 percent of young children in Iceland participated. Fruit and vegetable consumption at retail outlets went up 22 percent, and soda use went down 16 percent—for the first month, anyway. Considered the shining model of how to address childhood obesity, Scheving was awarded the Nordic Public Health Prize in 2004.[8]

However, the most recent childhood obesity data from Iceland shows that long-term obesity trends were not affected at all by the campaign. In fact, childhood obesity rates in Iceland rose 35 percent between 1990 and 2014. It now has the second highest obesity rate in Europe.[9] What about the rates of public obesity *stigma* in Iceland?

They are extremely high too, at least according to the preliminary data we collected there in 2011 and again in 2017.

The problem with the *LazyTown* campaign from the start was that the entire enterprise was based on the shared *belief* that more exercise and more fruit and vegetables lead to weight loss. The science just doesn't show that is true, though. The only interventions that seem to have any lasting impact on individual weight are highly *personalized* ones with considerable amounts of social and other practical support given to individuals. Unfortunately, even a good chunk of those fail as well. So, starting yoga programs or handing out oranges to children and expecting a noticeable drop in body mass index (BMI) as an outcome is a recipe for failure and frustration, regardless of how well-funded or engaging the idea.

The most we can realistically hope for with anti-obesity strategies that sidestep the scientific evidence is that they do no harm. This is why the disgust-focused campaigns being rolled out globally are especially concerning. New York City's Department of Health and Mental Hygiene decided shock would be the best approach in their 2009 anti-obesity campaign. Billboard and video ads showed liquid fat being poured or drunk from a soda can with the message "Don't drink yourself fat." Western Australia's Department of Health funded the LiveLighter campaign, which highlighted the unhealthiness of visible body fat using a "grabbable gut" tagline alongside pictures of internal organs ravaged by fat.[10] Mexican posters say, "No one dreams of becoming an overweight adult," implying that to end up fat is a wasted life. In the United Kingdom, legislators proposed labeling junk foods with pictures of bodies damaged by obesity, just like what had been done with the damaged body parts of smokers that appear on cigarette box labels.[11]

Do as We Say

Governments also sometimes legislate what people can eat or how they should behave, which has been strongly influenced by the success of anti-smoking efforts.[12] Making smoking illegal in public spaces, requiring dire health warning on cigarette boxes, and "sin-taxing" have driven mammoth reductions in smoking over the last several decades. Similar strategies for obesity are being tried around the world. Such strategies pass the costs of implementation onto food producers or consumers, so they are politically highly desirable.

Tactics that have been tried include penalizing obese employees by making them pay more for health insurance, taxing soda and junk food, and requiring warning labels on unhealthy food. The USDA (US Department of Agriculture), for example, states that food labeling is a "mechanism for consumers to make better dietary *choices* and thus increase their own and society's welfare."[13] The goal of such approaches remains fixed on consumer choice (rather than system-wide interventions).

The often-incorrect assumption that consumers are ignorant about which foods are fattening is also a common feature in these interventions. For childhood obesity in particular, the blame is generally placed on caregivers, especially mothers. Consider the World Health Organization's strategy which states, "Unlike most adults, children and adolescents cannot choose the environment in which they live or the food they eat. They also have a limited ability to understand the long-term consequences of their behavior. They therefore require special attention when fighting the obesity epidemic."[14]

Puerto Rico's government was debating a bill that would have schools identify overweight children and then provide monitored diet and exercise programs that would cost parents hundreds of dollars in fines if their child doesn't lose weight. Similarly, Children's Healthcare of Atlanta's Strong4Life campaign against childhood obesity in the United States included billboards rife with parent-blaming slogans such as, "Fat prevention begins at home and the buffet line." Australian anti-obesity campaigns went straight for the punch with the line, "Child obesity is child abuse." Posters from Israel show the naked stomach of a fat child, telling parents that fat is making their child depressed.

One of the most extreme mother-blaming anti-obesity policies has been rolled out in New Zealand.[15] There, the chief science advisor to the prime minister has been knighted for his world-class research showing that mothers' diet, stress levels, and weight shape the growing fetus' risk of obesity and chronic disease later in life.[16] His policy interpretation of these findings has become fully ingrained in government spending decisions. Money previously allocated to community-based interventions is being redirected onto behavior change for obese, pregnant women.

All obese, pregnant women in New Zealand are now targeted and treated as "high risk." They are then subjected to increased testing and surveillance under the state's control, regardless of the mothers' actual health status. New Zealand's approach monitors and manages women, rather than treating them as partners in creating better health for their children. It also ignores women's personal choices of how to manage their own pregnancies or births.

New Zealand excludes obese women from state-funded fertility treatments on the basis that their wombs are not safe for babies, a policy that pregnancy experts call arbitrary and unjust.[17] This policy has a socially exclusionary effect, since obesity rates are highest in low-income and Māori and Pacific Islanders. Once again, the more vulnerable socioeconomic groups carry the undue burden of these stigma-driven policies.

Doing the Opposite of What Was Intended

Policing pregnant women's weight causes them to worry that their weight is harming their unborn babies.[18] Instead of experiencing pregnancy as a time of joy and hope, pregnant women subjected to these fat interventions feel doubt, frustration, worry, powerlessness, and guilt. Once born, the children then carry the stigma. Interviews with New Zealand children show they also understand *they* are partly to blame for being fat, as they attributed not exercising enough to their own laziness.[19]

Globally, public health interventions around obesity seem to be having these same negative impacts on mental health and well-being. A study of Canadian adolescents compared how they reacted to various public service announcement posters from the United States, Australia, the United Kingdom, and Canada.[20] One such poster showed an overweight woman in a pink bathing suit with a line drawn along her body showing her body at a smaller size, with the tagline, "Started going for short walks during lunch hour."[21] Viewing the ad made people immediately anxious.

A recent analysis of public health obesity prevention campaigns showed that exposure to weight-focused obesity messages seemed to encourage people to want to change unhealthy behaviors. But the same exposure also decreased people's reporting of their "self-efficacy" or ability to make behavior changes compared to campaigns that didn't mention weight at all.[22] Food warning labels—which list calorie, fat, carbohydrate, and other nutritional content—seem to impose a "psychic tax" by generating shame and fear.[23] We also suspect those mother-blaming messages in New Zealand probably do little to help women keep their stress levels down during pregnancy. This stress, of course, can be treated as more evidence that the mothers are not providing an "optimal womb environment."

Even the very use of the term "obesity" can provoke judgmental feelings and drive anxiety. In our first round of interviews with 202 Arizona State University students, we had them list all of the words they could think of relevant to describing larger body sizes.[24] There were twenty-one commonly given words, including "fat" and "obese," as well as such variants as "chubby," "plump," "hefty," "unfit," and "high BMI." Then we organized these and had a further sample of 243 students categorize the list of twenty-one terms based upon which terms were most and least acceptable to use when talking with a friend about someone else, or to have a friend, healthcare provider, or stranger direct toward you if commenting on your weight. It proved that being labeled as "obese" was just as unwanted as being called "fat." In the more detailed interviews with a subset of students that followed, we were able to isolate that being labeled with "obesity" not only suggested you are socially unacceptable (which provides at least the option of saying "so what?") but *also* that you are dangerously unhealthy and a threat to public health. So, it seems to be difficult to design large-scale, *obesity* campaigns that don't perpetuate stigma and judgment.

Trying to Get It Right

Can anti-obesity efforts work better if they actively avoid stigma? In 2009, the United Kingdom launched a huge and expensive, social-marketing campaign called Change4Life. It purposefully avoided *any* use of the term "obesity" and eschewed images of overweight people. It talked of "fat in the body" rather than "fat bodies." But despite the good intentions, analyses suggest the campaign still created stigma damage. This may have been because the strategy focused on the need for decreases in weight; pounds lost was the marker of success. The conflicting messages generated—that fat is bad but fat is okay—were confusing and ultimately negative.[25] The campaign's lack of focus on "fat" also led to public debate over whether that was fat-shaming itself.

In the early years of Barack Obama's presidency, we sat down for an afternoon with chef Sam Kass. Kass was then director of Let's Move, US First Lady Michelle Obama's signature, long-running, child-focused anti-obesity campaign. Let's Move avoided talking about obesity and focused on health instead. It also included efforts to reduce anti-fat bullying. It was purposefully designed as an extremely kind campaign. Even so, it still focused on changing eating and exercise behavior, anchored on the importance of individual motivation. It also assumed that parents have at least some *control* over what happens to their children's weight. While Let's Move materials were scored by experts as less stigmatizing than other weight-focused public health efforts, their focus on helping overweight children continued to highlight them as the core problem.[26]

Legal scholar Paul Campos, a long-term critic of the "moral panic" that is generated by health efforts to tackle obesity, has passionately argued that Let's Move is yet another "particularly invidious form of bullying." Campos believes the anti-bullying angle itself is a problem, because it

> is in effect arguing that the way to stop the bullying of fat kids is to get rid of fat kids . . . [T]he profound shaming and stigmatization of fat children that is an inevitable product of the campaign's absurd premise that the bodies of heavier than average children are by definition defective, and that this "defect" can be cured through lifestyle changes . . . [F]at kids have enough problems without the additional burden of being subjected to government-approved pseudo-scientific garbage about how they could be thin if they just ate their vegetables and played outside more often.[27]

To paraphrase, anti-obesity campaigns are fueling the stigma fire. Framing obesity as a public health problem that requires action to change people's bad lifestyle choices creates powerful moral overtones about how people should behave. A thin body is implied or expressed as the primary, sometimes only, sign of health and good citizenship.[28] In this way, efforts to tackle obesity are perhaps the most powerful and influential factor affecting how people globally see both their health and their bodies.[29]

Poverty Complicates Everything

Another related challenge is that anti-obesity strategies that embrace individual behavior change assume that everyone has the opportunity, capacity, and capability to make "healthy choices." This is especially problematic in the poorest communities. Choice is diminished by lack of available resources such as money, time, public amenities, or information. People who are struggling to make ends meet often feel they don't have many choices about anything.

Consider the efforts to improve the quality of food consumed as a means to improve population health. People are not just choosing foods based on taste preference but also household schedules and economics. Purchased high fat, sugar, and sodium meals are often cheaper, and easier to access, for people with limited means or time. For example, Alex, along with Cindi SturtzSreetharan, has recently been working on a study of how middle-class Japanese commuters in Osaka, Japan, navigate their anxieties around an overwhelming array of outlets selling delicious foods as they traverse the city twice each day. Similarly, in many lower-income urban neighborhoods of higher-income countries, fast-food options tend to dominate and can provide cheaper and faster family meals than can be produced through home cooking. (Notably, some studies have found that these "food swamps" predict higher neighborhood obesity rates and/or worse nutrition, others have not.)[30] Perhaps more importantly, "fast-food bans," like the one enacted in South Los Angeles to control the density of fast-food outlets, do not seem to reduce obesity and may even increase it.[31]

Raising the cost of these convenience or processed foods or controlling fast-food outlets as a means to dissuade purchases may or may not work, but it seems to negatively impact lower-income households. And there are other ways discrimination or lower power can block access to healthier food for such vulnerable groups. When we were doing interviews with Latinx households in South Phoenix, Arizona, in 2008 in the wake of new anti-immigrant legislation, people explained to us that travel to supermarkets to buy healthier, cheaper food had become too risky. For undocumented people, Arizona traffic stops could lead to detention or deportation. It was much safer to buy closer to home, in more expensive, less healthy, neighborhood corner stores.

In low-income households, sometimes food isn't just about having enough to eat, either; it can be about how people eat together. We have seen this firsthand, over and over, in our own research. For example, take a study Alex did in the mid-1990s to understand how parents in the American Southeast organized their children's meals. She was working in rural Washington-Wilkes County, Georgia, a region with extremely high rates of overweight in an already overweight part of the country. Diabetes rates were off the charts, which is why we were invited to work in the town. Walmart had recently opened a mega store around twenty miles out of town, which meant all the town's local supermarkets had been shuttered. The county had been turned into a classic rural "food desert."[32]

Washington-Wilkes parents, many of whom worked long hours at minimum wage, had little *time* to plan meals, travel to shop, and home cook food. This meant they had to rely on packaged and convenience foods or takeout. Moreover, having to work so hard to support their families meant that the little time they had together was precious. The one time each day everyone connected was over dinner. When the team surveyed eighty-nine parents of 3-to-6-year-old children in the one preschool in the county, and then did in-depth interviews about children's food, eating, and weight with nine of the parents.[33] In the surveys, parents were able to identify correctly what a healthy preschool diet should be, but what the children were eating was, on average, much higher in calories—with a mean of 2,025 calories a day—than what is recommended as appropriate for preschool children (1,400–1,600 calories per day). Interviews made it clearer what was happening: The most important thing for these families was for everyone to be together over dinner each evening, enjoying each other's company and the food. Taking time away to cook and clean dishes or spending time fighting with the kids to eat their broccoli undermined the family's experience of togetherness. On the other hand, bringing home (high calorie) takeout made sense: it was cheap, quick, and close; no need to spend time prepping a meal; and everyone enjoyed it. If parents cooked, they tended to favor a traditional southern-style meal, also highly caloric but appealing and meaningful to everyone eating it.[34]

Campaigns that focus on individual behavior change often forget that people live with and want and need to relate to other people. Nutrition isn't the only thing people consider when they decide what to eat: cost, accessibility, time, preference, family, and identity all factor in, too. Poverty complicates the notion that all "healthy" choices are the best ones for families. Similarly, "fat taxes" are implemented with the goal of changing what people purchase by making junk foods less attractive. Extreme poverty complicates this simple formula, but no one seems to be considering exactly how. We suspect such strategies also become shaming, and often counterproductive, when they play out in real-world communities where poverty severely reduces people's purchasing options.[35] Mexico is a good case study to think about how this could happen.

Downstream Effects: The Sweet Case of Mexico

Obesity rates are sky-high in Mexico, and diabetes is a leading cause of death. According to one study published right before the national anti-obesity strategy was implemented in the 2000s, these rates were predicted to push direct healthcare costs up by US$1 billion.[36] Diabetes treatments cost something like $800 per person per annum and they are particularly burdensome on healthcare systems because diabetes is a lifelong condition. Mexico also has the world's highest per capita consumption of sweetened beverages at 0.4 liters per person daily, more than 20 percent of the average calorie requirement (figure 6.1).[37]

The Mexican government responded to this situation with one of the most comprehensive, centralized anti-obesity initiatives in the world, the National Agreement for Healthy Nutrition (ANSA).[38] ANSA targets people's intake of sweetened drinks as public health enemy number one in the Mexican war on obesity and diabetes.[39]

Phase 1 of the ANSA campaign was to raise public awareness of obesity and related chronic diseases, emphasizing the importance of making good diet and exercise choices.[40] The public were told through national media campaigns: "Don't harm yourself drinking sugary drinks" and "Soft drinks are sweet. Diabetes is not." Community-level education efforts included a spandex-suited Mexican *Lucha Libre* wrestler "wrestling against obesity" to demonstrate healthy lifestyle choices.[41] In parallel to this campaign, the *Alianza por la Salud Alimentaria* (Alliance for Healthy Food), funded by the anti-tobacco World Lung Foundation, launched a campaign in 2015 implying that parents are abusive when they allow their children sweet drinks. In true parent-blaming fashion, they asked, "What did your children eat today?"

Phase 2 of the ANSA campaign added new "sin taxes."[42] In 2013, Mexican President Peña Nieto proposed a 10 percent tax on all soda. Multinational corporations like Coca-Cola pushed back, suggesting that the tax was part of a global conspiracy led by New York Mayor Michael Bloomberg. As a result, *Ley Antiobesided*, enacted in 2014, placed a much less punitive 1 peso (<1 cent) per liter tax on all sweetened beverages (except juice). It also introduced an 8 percent tax on the highest energy (junk snack) foods.

Evidence suggests that soda consumption in Mexico is down a little from the high of 172 liters per capita drunk in 2011. The decrease was highest in the lowest income households at around 9 percent.[43] However, there isn't any evidence yet that this decrease is doing anything to lower obesity rates *per se*. The government has happily raked in the additional revenue nonetheless (70 billion pesos as of mid-2017, according to the finance ministry). Some of the income is supposedly slated to be used to improve drinking water access in Mexican schools.[44]

So, on the surface, these efforts have brought some success for some stakeholders. But understanding the impact of stigma on health requires us to always look at the downstream effects. This case, therefore, gives us an opportunity to think through how we might *anticipate* and *predict* the possible negative outcomes of weight-focused global health interventions. In particular, we can make a best guess at how these national efforts might inadvertently hurt the poorest and the most vulnerable. But first, we need a little background.

In Chiapas, in southern Mexico, Coca-Cola consumption is probably the highest in the world. According to anthropologist Jaime Tomás Page Pliego, one village he was working consumed on average 2.25 liters per person daily.[45] This translates to about half of the daily average calories needed, without contributing any protein or other basic nutrients. Why are these consumption rates so high here? The answer lies in how Coca-Cola has become so embedded in everyday life. It is used as a gift around important events, like betrothals and birthdays. It is used in Catholic church services in place of wine.

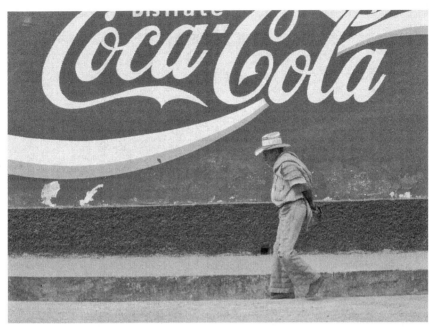

Figure 6.1. Advertising Coca-Cola in San Cristóbal, Chiapas, Mexico. © Alamy

Drinking soda is also tied to other aspects of stigma in complex and subtle ways. In the late 1990s, we conducted a detailed study of 8-to-12-year-old children living in the tumbled, dusty informal settlements around the small city of Xalapa in central-east Mexico. We observed how the poorest households dealt with money shortages by gradually cutting out more and more foods until homemade tortillas were the only food left.[46] Eating *only* tortillas was considered to be humiliating as it showed others the depth of your poverty.

Serving soda helped offset this shame. The extra calories also helped you feel full. So, the cheapest, socially acceptable family meal that could fill you was a pile of homemade tortillas and a large bottle of soda. Moreover, when visitors (like the anthropologists) came to your house, offering soda was the most cost-effective way to show hospitality. A huge bottle of water from a tap simply did not fill this same social need.[47] Similarly, in Amber's recent fieldwork doing participant observation and interviewing women in Paraguay, she confirmed that offering an off-brand soda was considered by some to be a sign of poverty or poor taste—a reason for others, who are only slightly less poor, to mock or refuse the gift.

Given this context, when a sin tax is introduced, poor people are still socially obligated to buy and give Coca-Cola—now it just costs more. Not buying Coke just because the price went up is not an option when the underlying social obligations remain.[48] In such communities, the new taxes add to the already long list of intersecting economic and social exclusions already faced by those living on the margins of society. As this example shows, we can reliably predict that the negative effects of direct or indirect stigma as a public health tool always tend to run downhill, onto the poorest, the most excluded, and the most stigmatized communities.

What we expect will happen next, if the handwashing and cigarette smoking examples that we discussed in part I are anything to go by, is that drinking soda will soon become a stigmatized index of ignorance and poverty. People who drink Coke will be viewed like those who smoke cigarettes or don't wash their hands. And, indeed, we have heard one parent from Latin America say of another—upon viewing a toddler drinking soda out of a bottle—"I just don't feel comfortable arranging a play date with that child's family. I mean, they give the baby soda in a bottle. We clearly don't share the same values."

Globally, too, this shift appears to be happening in the public health industry. A recent public health assessment of what to do about sugar-sweetened drink consumption in South Africa ended with the ominous recommendation that, "One important task is to ensure greater public awareness of the harmfulness of sugar . . . Sugar should be portrayed as the 'new tobacco.'"[49] And that brings us full circle, right back to where we started at the beginning of this book.

What Next?

So, what's next for weight stigma? Our planet will continue to get fatter for some time yet. Given the rising costs of healthcare, the threats of the "obesity epidemic" are going to keep governments panicking. Anti-obesity strategies and media coverage of obesity as a public threat will continue to intensify anti-obesity discourse, education, and activity.

More people will be in the way of inescapable public stigma. And unless we completely overhaul our public health strategies for tackling obesity, they will continue to cause the stigmatizing *shame* and *blame*. Weight will continue to grow as an emotional issue. It will depress people even further. The culmination of all of these efforts will likely *promote*, not discourage, weight gain.

For people who work to deliver health, what can be done? There doesn't seem any easy way to remove the powerful "fat as bad" message that is so encoded in almost every aspect of modern, digital life. Regardless, constant attention to how obesity programs and campaigns are framed is vital. We especially need a constant and critical analysis of the infiltration of blaming messages.[50]

Campaigns that avoid a direct focus on obesity, instead promoting healthy lifestyles and self-esteem, are a sensible place to start. In many countries, the immediate and expensive health issue isn't actually obesity—it's diabetes. As a result, we suspect that there will be a shift in focus from obesity reduction to diabetes prevention. If historical cases of stigma prove true, this won't spell the end of the stigma but rather the stigma will be reshaped against diabetes. In places like India, where diabetes rates are extremely high, this process has already begun. Anthropologist Emily Mendenhall has found that diabetic adults in Delhi are starting to cope with growing stigmas by focusing on the nonmedical meanings of diabetes.[51] This reduces their emotional stress and risk of depression but also erodes their self-care and likelihood of seeking medical support.

The effort to remove individual stigmas one-by-one really is an uphill battle. We need health professionals to be more aware of intersecting and layering stigmas. We need to think about designing obesity interventions in ways that unlock and release stigma. For example, let's say the goal is to reduce diabetes in a low-income town in

Latin America where soda consumption is extremely high and water security is very low. A stigma-free solution is to provide taps or fountains for drinking water in schools and other public places. This approach addresses an underlying structural problem (water access), gives people an easy health-promoting solution (drink water), and possibly supports obesity destigmatization (omitting the mention of obesity).[52]

Even if such an approach doesn't always work, at the very least it does no harm. Like with handwashing, no amount of behavior stigmatization is going to work if people don't have access to the basic infrastructure they need (toilets and taps) to make healthier choices. By insisting on this approach, we are likely to create new stigmas and risk profiles. Stigma-free solutions tend to be about designing better infrastructure and more equitable societies. Such solutions are also the ones that have the best chance of working. A stigma-free public health strategy is much better at creating real and sustainable solutions.

As a first step, what matters most for dealing with fat stigma is rendering it more *visible*. The seeming invisibility of stigma to everyone that matters—policy makers, health educators, friends, family, and self—is what makes it truly dangerous in this context. Compare the invisibility of fat stigma to the in-your-face, hypervisibility of obesity prevention efforts right now. We need to become aware and attuned to the reality that fat stigma is a second globalizing epidemic.

The rapid growth of fat stigma, completely globalized within a decade, also shows we need to be tracking real-time *changes* in stigma. This will require us to develop and apply better tools for a public health of *stigma epidemiology*. A regularized, systematic means to test for generalized weight-related stigma within and between populations would be a great start. This would help identify and highlight concerning trends, while also explicating the conditions—social, economic, and otherwise—where fat stigma is most damaging. It would also allow us to build, then test, anti-obesity and other public health efforts that—at the very least—do no harm.

The Bottom Line

Public health approaches to obesity prevention are seeded with stigmatizing notions of individual responsibility and blame. Anti-obesity campaigns initiated across the globe are contributing to growing fat stigma. We can't say conclusively what effective, non-stigmatizing campaigns look like, because we are not yet tracking the relevant measures of stigma. To fight the global, compounded impacts on almost every aspect of human health, we need to galvanize efforts that make stigma visible.

Part III

Crazy

7

Once Crazy, Always Crazy

Clara was born in the early 1930s in New Zealand, a doctor's daughter. In her teens, she had been a rising track and field star. Photos of her show a stunning, tall blond soaring above the high jump bar in the 1950 British Empire Games (figure 7.1). However, the family tells the story of how she couldn't handle the pressure of the competition, or the transition to university that happened about the same time. She "broke down" and became disorganized, dirty, confused, withdrawn, and agitated. Despite everyone's best efforts to set her up with jobs and dates, she repeatedly proved both unemployable and unmarriageable. She "refused" and "defied" the medical treatments organized by her father. She was "crazy Clara," "unstable," "selfish," "demanding," "unwanted," and—most of all—"useless" and "an embarrassment." Family would say she needed to "just snap out of it," "grow up," "behave herself," and "stop being so darn self-involved."

Clara's medical records show a life of chaos and confusion, of numerous doctors, institutions, diagnoses, and treatments. She was diagnosed on and off with schizophrenia and bipolar depression, both very disabling conditions. At that time, effective modern treatments for such serious mental illness were in their infancy. For Clara, there were years of electroshock therapy and other years of forced injections of long-acting antipsychotic drugs. She was given a cascade of different prescriptions with notations about her complaints of intolerable side effects. Pages upon pages of medical notes swam with a sense of her isolation and confusion. When she died in 2006, the email informing the family read, "It's . . . difficult to think what was in Clara's life that can be celebrated. It has been the saddest life I have ever known." Even in death, it proved hard for those who knew her best to place any value on her life even in retrospect; her entire life was pitied and seen as wasted.

These views of Clara's life illustrate the social devaluation that often accompanies severe mental illness. Of all mental illnesses, schizophrenia is one of the most debilitating and the most stigmatized. As a result, it is also one of the best conditions to study why destigmatization is crucial for effective medical treatment. In this chapter, we'll use the term "people diagnosed with schizophrenia," or PDWS for short. The fact that this term even *exists* is the result of long, hard work by antistigma activists. As we've tried to show—and as the terminology around

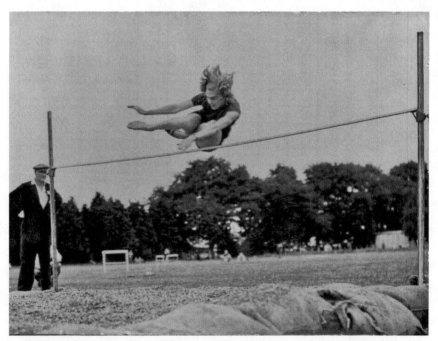

Figure 7.1. Clara competing in the high jump in the 1950 Commonwealth Games in Christchurch, New Zealand. Photo provided by A. Brewis

mental health so clearly demonstrates—language is one of the very important frontlines for people fighting against stigma.

Schizophrenia affects some twenty-five million people globally, and, as it did for Clara, it typically emerges in early adulthood. A debilitating brain condition with both genetic and environmental triggers, schizophrenia distorts how people think and relate to the world around them. People with untreated schizophrenia find it difficult to distinguish real from imagined and to function within society. Expressing emotion, like smiling, in social settings becomes a trial. Their off-kilter behaviors make observers uncomfortable or scared, as they seem confused, talk oddly, and don't show the appropriate sympathy for others' suffering. Untreated, they can find it especially hard to maintain relationships, parent effectively, or manage work. Medical treatment is clearly needed and warranted.

Being labeled schizophrenic elicits particular fear. This fear is partly a result of movies and stories that paint PDWS as homicidal maniacs. However, the evidence suggests something quite different. PDWS are much more likely to be victims than perpetrators of violent crime. As one British PDWS commented, "If it's on the news or TV it's usually because they've brandished a sword on the high street or attacked someone. There's never a story about a schizophrenic who saves [the] life of granny who falls in canal."[1]

Stigma around schizophrenia also stems from the widely held belief that it is untreatable; essentially: once crazy, always crazy. Certainly, a large proportion of people institutionalized in mental health facilities are PDWS. But with treatment, a full and lasting recovery is possible in half of cases and about a third completely recover. Even in full recovery, though, people diagnosed with schizophrenia must still battle with stigma. Studies in high-income countries show that even fully treated PDWS are not trusted in positions of authority, as friends, or as partners.[2] Because of the fear their diagnosis elicits, they find it hard to connect socially, get good jobs, or rent housing. People don't want them near children. These forms of active discrimination push them toward underemployment and unemployment, homelessness, and poverty. These conditions in turn worsen mental illness, because they reduce access to services, undermine consistency in treatment, and generally stress people out.

The basic key to successful treatment of schizophrenia is starting early and sticking with it. Many patients only need outpatient medication. But even in the high-income countries like the United States, half of those with noticeable symptoms never seek medical treatment at all.[3] People with early warning symptoms like unusual thoughts or odd speech may retreat into denial or adopt a deep sense of futility. Their families often follow suit.

Even if they do seek medical help, people with schizophrenia report they are poorly treated, and they aren't imagining it. Consider a study that compared PDWS in a large government hospital in Hong Kong to people in the same facility being treated for diabetes. The PDWS dealt with rude hospital staff and excessive use of physical and chemical restraints. They were given less information about their treatment and side effects and had more infringements of their patients' rights.[4] Not surprisingly, they often didn't show up to subsequent scheduled clinic visits.

The stigma of schizophrenia can also worsen the symptoms that patients are experiencing. One study of PDWS in fourteen European countries found that people who were exposed to more stigmatized reactions from others had worse hallucinations and were more likely to develop other problems like depression.[5] Hearing constantly that you are useless, dangerous, or incompetent means it is hard to even trust yourself and your own treatment decisions. It can make you wary of reaching out to those with the same condition or who understand it in ways that could provide real emotional support. Why would you connect to others labeled as "crazies" if you, too, believe they are dangerous and unpredictable?[6]

Schizophrenia is a relatively rare, serious mental illness that affects some 1–2 percent of people. But something like a quarter of us will grapple with some significant mental health challenge at some point in our lives.[7] Mental illness is a catch-all category that also includes autism, attention-deficit disorder, learning disabilities, depression, and eating disorders. Yet, despite how common it is, all mental illness is highly stigmatized. Crazy. Loony. Mad. Mental. Nuts. Even children can list more than 250 disparaging terms for someone with mental illness,[8] each of which resonates with a sense of danger, disability, violence, incapacity, untreatability, unwantedness, and loneliness. It is common for people living with schizophrenia to report that these stigmatizing ideas, and the fear and rejection they evoke, are more distressing and disabling than the mental illness itself. Stigma damages mental health because it unravels our most valued, core social identities. It fundamentally diminishes who we are.

Consider Zoe, a British woman who has been diagnosed with posttraumatic stress disorder (PTSD), depression, and anxiety. Her doctors told her to take a leave of absence from her job, but she knew she enjoyed it, knew she was good at it, and wanted to stay working. Unfortunately, her colleagues found out about her illness. They called her "mad" and "difficult" and "griefy." She saw emails they sent making fun of her. One day, removing something from her handbag, her supervisor asked jokingly if she was pulling out a weapon. The constant negative attention from coworkers took a toll on both her physical and mental health. She was forced to give up the job she loved. She said, "I can cope with work despite my mental health problems, but not with all this discrimination, hostility, bullying, and harassment . . . This trauma from work caused me such immense despair and lack of hope . . . My question is this: Is my life any less valuable than my supervisor's or colleagues' because I have mental health problems and they don't?"[9]

To avoid pain and rejection, people like Clara and Zoe may hide and deny their mental health condition from others, worsening or extending their illness. Or they, quite understandably, may avoid seeking treatment at all. This damage created by public stigma toward those with mental illness is widely appreciated and understood by the mental health profession. In fact, destigmatization has long been a major element of global mental health promotion efforts. But despite decades of hard work, the removal of sustained stigma around mental illness has proven elusive. This section explains why, and what we can do about it.

Goffman, Stigma, and Labels

None of this is news to modern mental health practitioners. They know that stigma can impede and undermine effective mental illness treatment in the clinic and out in the community. That's why fighting stigma is at the heart of modern public health approaches to mental wellness. Much of this current thought about why destigmatizing is critical to mental health treatment stems from sociologist Erving Goffman's writing in the 1960s.[10] Goffman understood what stigma felt like in the most personal terms. Growing up in provincial Canada in the 1920s and 1930s, he was the only son of a Russian immigrant. He was Jewish in a town with no other Jewish families, and—perhaps most painfully—he was very short.[11] He was dreadfully teased and bullied as a child.

Possibly as a result of this childhood, Goffman's first academic work, based on two years of fieldwork in the small, isolated Scottish Shetland Islands, tackled the idea of how people act constantly in their daily lives to avoid humiliation.[12] He hung out at the island's only hotel, attended socials in the community hall, and talked with small-scale sheep farmers, fishermen, and their wives. But mostly, he observed what people did when they were together. He decided that the ways that people interacted were mostly shaped by their efforts to ensure they weren't embarrassed or didn't embarrass others. To him, the daily rituals of social interaction—how people presented themselves— were all complex efforts to avoid shame.

Goffman's next long-term ethnographic fieldwork took him directly to what was then the heart of modern mental illness treatment: the psychiatric hospitals around Washington, DC. For three years, he worked in the wards, followed doctors on rounds, and talked to patients. The resulting book, *Asylums* (1961), was a powerful indictment of the institutional treatment of mental health patients at the time.[13] Comparing the clinical staff to guards and the patients to inmates in concentration camps, he explained how the daily rituals of the asylum didn't work to treat or cure patients but rather taught patients to behave in ways that made them easier for caretakers to manage

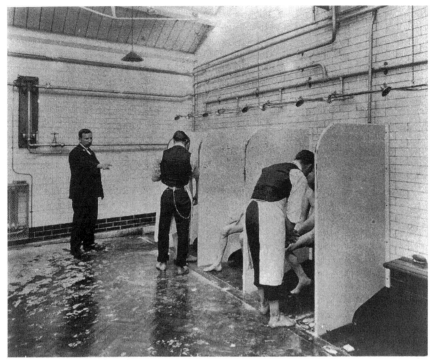

Figure 7.2. Male patients being washed on admission to Long Grove Asylum, United Kingdom, circa 1930s. From the Wellcome Collection, https://wellcomecollection.org/

(figure 7.2). Psychiatrists, to Goffman, were part of the problem, because patients' compliance was valued over a cure for their condition. Their words and actions also reinforced the idea that people institutionalized with mental illness were incurable, which then became self-fulfilling.

Goffman's work and other studies around this time explained that mental illness could be created by the diagnosis itself.[14] Labeling someone with a mental disorder, they argued, leads people to self-identify with the attached moral messages and stereotypes. Their behavior then conforms with the label. Following this argument, then, people diagnosed with schizophrenia become incompetent, unpredictable, violent, and dangerous because society tells them that is what is expected and normal for someone with their condition.[15] Goffman's concise 1964 book *Stigma* identified that stigma is at the core of how mental illness is constructed and why treatment fails.[16] The single most influential sociological text ever published, *Stigma* described the constant, draining work that stigmatized people have to do as they strive to present themselves to others as normal.[17] To Goffman, this only contributed to the progression of mental illness, which he considered to be, fundamentally, a social construction, not an inescapable biological fact. In other words, Goffman realized that labeling someone crazy is a product of consensus, and stigma is at the heart. This was progressive thinking at the time, and by the 1970s, mental health efforts caught up.[18]

Removing Mental Illness Stigma

Thanks to Goffman and his colleagues, stigma reduction has been a key part of mental health campaigns for half a century. Different strategies are now commonly applied, most of which are focused on changing the attitudes of the general public toward mental illness. These efforts roughly sort into five types: relabeling the illness itself, reframing how people see the causes of illness, educating the general public or health professionals to build empathy, connecting people socially to build empathy, and supporting anti-stigma activism. So, what have we learned about the best ways to destigmatize effectively? Surprisingly little, it turns out—and not for lack of trying on all five fronts.

Relabel

If Goffman and his colleagues were right that labeling is the core of the problem, then the simplest fix is to rename mental illnesses with terms that remove judgment and shame. Words are used that communicate the biological basis for the condition and that imply its curability. For example, schizophrenia has variously been renamed "dopamine dysregulation disorder," "integration disorder," "youth onset cognitive and reality distortion," and "salience syndrome."[19]

Relabeling is a great idea in theory. In reality, the problem seems to be that a new label is still a label and fear is still fear.[20] In Japan, an advocacy group of relatives of PDWS pushed for a replacement of the established term for schizophrenia: *seishin bunretsu byo* ("mind-split disease"). The label conjured up images of extreme violence and the impossibility of recovery. The term was so bad that only 7 percent of Japanese psychiatrists said they habitually used the term with their patients. In 2002, schizophrenia was renamed *togo shitcho sho* ("integration disorder"). This made psychiatrists more comfortable with sharing the diagnosis with patients, and patients were more optimistic that they could be successfully treated.[21] Since this name change, newspaper coverage of violence associated with schizophrenia seems to have gone down. But, at the same time, coverage of violence associated with bipolar disorder seems to have gone up. This suggests one wrinkle in the renaming strategy: The threat of violence associated with severe mental illness may just transfer to a different severe condition in the public imagination.[22]

To combat this problem, a recent effort is to relabel mental illness as part of a continuum of brain types. This "neurodiversity" effort is based on neuro-cognitive research that suggests brain disorders might confer some advantages, too.[23] For example, people diagnosed with autism spectrum disorder (ASD) may process system information like computer languages or mathematics more effectively than others.[24] Dyslexia seems to allow clearer 3D visualization, which could lead to better performance in tasks like computer graphics. Attention-deficit/hyperactivity disorder (ADHD) allows for creativity, and hyper focus, and the types of peripheral acuity that may be useful for emergency responders.[25]

The label of "neurodiversity" promotes brain diversity as being good for society, just like biodiversity is good for ecosystems.[26] Some companies like HP Enterprises and Microsoft have started hiring programs to recruit a neurodiverse workforce, with the argument that it is not only socially responsible but may also help their bottom lines.[27] There isn't much evidence of whether this approach is working yet, because there haven't been many studies. But because the neurodiversity push works to destigmatize through positive messaging, at least it (like good renaming) probably isn't doing too much damage.

Reframe

The prevailing post-Goffman wisdom in psychology is that mental illness is shaped—but not completely determined—by its negative social labels.[28] This suggests that public stigma still socializes people diagnosed with schizophrenia to expect they will be mistreated and rejected. In turn, they then feel more stigma from people around them. Their efforts to cope (e.g., withdrawing from others, hiding treatment, or educating others) then damage their jobs, social connections, and self-esteem. This view remains highly influential in social science and suggests that changing public beliefs and self-stigma are crucially important.

Currently, the vast majority of stigma interventions focus on reframing or changing public perceptions of mental illness. Since stigma is often about blame, much effort has focused on reframing public perceptions about the causes of mental illness. Theoretically, if people believe problems are "medical" in origin rather than due to a bad choice or weakness of character, they might reduce their blame of the person and, thereby, reduce stigma.[29]

Unfortunately, reframing public perceptions to emphasize the medical aspects of mental illness doesn't help as much as hoped. Compared with fifty years ago, a much greater proportion of the public today perceives that genes play a role in causing schizophrenia. Telling people that mental illness is a disease "like any other" does reduce some notions of blame. However, the level of rejection toward people with mental illness seems to have gone up, not down, over time.[30]

In 1990 and 2001, German researchers read people vignettes that described the clinical signs of schizophrenia, without naming the condition. They asked participants to tell them what they thought was the cause of the listed symptoms. Popular answers focused on stressful life events, stress at work, broken homes, lack of willpower, and immoral lifestyles. Biological and hereditary explanations of the disordered behaviors increased markedly over the studied decade, indicating an increase in public perceptions of medical causality.

But it turned out that a reframed medical understanding of schizophrenia didn't make people less stigmatizing—especially in the ways that would really matter. Participants said they still didn't want to rent a room or live next door to people with these symptoms.[31] In addition, it seems that the focus on medical and genetic aspects of mental illness also makes people less optimistic about long-term prognosis, reinforcing the idea that those who are sick are also dangerous.[32]

For these reasons, the reframing approach does not often seem to work well as a destigmatization effort. Moreover, there is some evidence that reframing may shift stigma from traits that are perceived as less permanent or durable categories (e.g., stress, willpower, immorality) to traits that are perceived as more permanent or durable (e.g., genetics, incurable medical conditions). In doing so, reframing efforts may even do more harm than good.

Reeducate

So, what about direct efforts at public education by increasing knowledge about what living with the condition is like for people? These approaches, strongly influenced by social psychology, assume stigma is rooted in learned ignorance and prejudiced stereotypes. As a result, if people acquire better information about a condition, replacing misinformation with facts, then stigma should be reduced (e.g., "PDWS are more likely to be victims than perpetrators of violence"). These approaches are often adopted because they are relatively cheap and easy. The effects of these types of interventions, however, seem to be mostly transitory.[33]

One of the very first campaigns was the brainchild of Canadian sociologist Elaine Cumming. For six months in 1951–1952, she and her husband plastered a small prairie town community with radio spots, brochures, and school visits. The key message was "What we define as normal is relative." Unfortunately, their energetic efforts had very little measured impact on public attitudes.[34] People's ideas of what was abnormal proved to be well-established and resisted adjustment.

Nonetheless, anti-stigma efforts have stuck with this same general approach since Cumming's campaign and the results have been much the same. For example, the Australian federal government spent millions on a national public advertising campaign to increase community awareness regarding mental illness.[35] They worked hard to monitor the impacts of the campaign (unlike most similar projects), so the results of their program evaluation are likely more reliable. The outcome was "no practical impact on community attitudes or behaviour towards people with mental illness, with consumers reporting that stigma and discrimination remained at the high level that existed prior."

One problem with the education approach is that there are so many other competing messages in the media that reinforce the idea that people diagnosed with schizophrenia and other mental health conditions are "not like us" and should be feared and avoided. However, public education efforts still don't seem to work well even when there is little media exposure.

In India, the SMART mental health anti-stigma effort included visiting forty-two remote villages. The anti-stigma education included a theater troupe, screening of a video of a person living with mental illness describing their experiences, and a well-known local actor discussing stigma. Moderated discussion followed. Immediately after the intervention, there was a measurable improvement in community members' disagreement with the statement that "people with mental illness cannot live a good, rewarding life." But there was no change at all in more fundamental views that "mentally ill people shouldn't get married" and "mentally ill people tend to be violent."[36] These are exactly the important public attitude changes that are needed for real improvement to people's daily lives.

There is a further fundamental flaw in focusing on changing the public: The worst stigma comes from health professionals. Time and time again, studies of patients with access to adequate psychiatric care highlight that the most damaging stigma for them is encountered inside the clinic once they seek medical help. Patients complain of feeling "experimented on" as psychiatrists manipulate the type and dosage of their drugs. They feel rejected when asked about their suicidality. They feel very emotionally disconnected from their doctors.[37]

Studies of psychiatrists and other people who manage mentally ill clients suggest their views are not much different from the public at large. For example, clinicians say they don't want to be friends with or otherwise hang out with mentally ill people, even if they treat them. Because of their professional positions, they hold more power than most to help or hurt, and sadly, studies show that clinicians are unaware of the systematically poor treatment the severely mentally ill receive while under their care. Their behavior is so ingrained as "business as usual" that it is often completely invisible to them. Such is the nature of institutionalized stigma.

As a result, some education efforts have focused, sensibly, on changing attitudes of the groups with the greatest ability, opportunity, and power to make a difference: future doctors. One example, the Education Not Discrimination intervention, was rolled out in four medical schools in England.[38] It included a short lecture about stigma and discrimination, had people with mental health challenges tell their stories, and had the students interact with actors playing patients and caregivers. Short-term outcomes seemed good; the students gained knowledge and exhibited more empathy. However, six months after the intervention, the improvements had all but disappeared. One explanation is that the students had started their psychiatric rotation in the interim. As soon as they had contact with real people with severe mental illness conditions, the stigma reemerged.[39]

Connect

Creating personal social connections is another approach, built on the idea that we are more sympathetic to those we get to know or feel we have things in common with.[40] This one-person-at-a-time approach has done well for addressing the stigma of people with physical disabilities. For example, meeting people in wheelchairs at social or sporting events can result in able-bodied people being willing to be closer to those with disabilities. Add a service dog and the smiles and positive interactions increase even more.[41] This empathy adjustment seems to work best when the people being targeted belong to social groups that are similar (e.g., in terms of class and race/ethnicity) to those experiencing stigma.[42]

This approach has been much less successful in reducing the stigma of severe mental illness compared to physical disabilities. For example, people who were given headphones so they could "hear" the auditory hallucinations associated with schizophrenia, reported feeling more empathy for PDWS, but they also wanted more social distance. And knowing people living with chronic and serious mental illness has not proven to be a recipe for building empathy.

In a study of people with mental illness in Hong Kong, some 60 percent of patients said their families assumed they were highly violent; more than half thought their families hated them.[43] One sister shouted, "Crazy people shouldn't live with normal ones! I'll sever any connection with you! If you don't move out, I'll just throw away all your belongings!"[44] Being more aware of serious differences can make people want to steer clear, not get closer. Consequently, these types of empathy interventions for severe mental illness can backfire, and experts suggest they should only be used with extreme caution.[45]

Advocate

Advocates work on behalf of stigmatized people to increase empathy and decrease stigma. Advocacy, not surprisingly, works best when there is a powerful, popular, and legitimate public face to it—someone that people already choose to listen to. Large, well-organized, public health anti-stigma campaigns know this well, and often use celebrities to garner attention, create empathy, and endorse the stigmatized condition as acceptable.

Celebrities can help normalize and give a sympathetic (and even pretty) face to a condition. Public figures' self-disclosure may encourage others to move into treatment. It can stimulate public debate and reflection, with the possibility of not only creating empathy but also improving legal protections or insurance coverage—things that really matter.

When US First Lady Betty Ford revealed she was in treatment for substance abuse in the 1970s, she was hailed as brave rather than weak. Suddenly, the idea of inpatient drug treatment (at least for wealthy, white women) became more acceptable. Similarly, when actor Brooke Shields revealed she was using medication for postpartum depression—and fellow actor Tom Cruise publicly lambasted her decision—it spurred public sympathy for Shields and helped normalize the condition. She was able to spread her message that, "If any good can come of Mr. Cruise's ridiculous rant, let's hope that it gives much-needed attention to a serious disease. Perhaps now is the time to call on doctors, particularly obstetricians and pediatricians, to screen for postpartum depression."[46]

Carrie Fisher, actor-writer of "Star Wars" fame, was diagnosed with bipolar disorder in her twenties.[47] She struggled with the mental illness and the associated stigma through much of her life. In 2008, she used her autobiography to advocate for a kinder way of understanding mental illness. She wrote, "living with manic depression takes a tremendous amount of balls. Not unlike a tour of duty in Afghanistan (though the bombs and bullets, in this case, come from the inside). At times, being bipolar can be an all-consuming challenge, requiring a lot of stamina and even more courage, so if you're living with this illness and functioning at all, it's something to be proud of, not ashamed of."

Such messages in part work because we feel we "know" celebrities and already feel intimately and positively connected to them. We would have them around to dinner if we could. Moreover, the media shows more kindness to celebrities with stigmatized conditions than other members of the public.[48] They are less likely to paint them as dangerous or stupid or useless. The version of mental illness or other disability or disease that is projected is often sanitized and, hence, much less threatening. Leonardo DiCaprio and David Beckham live with obsessive compulsive disorder. Adam Levine manages ADHD. Princess Diana and Elton John struggled with eating disorders. But all of these famous people look good and appear in full control of their lives, even as they cope "heroically" with their conditions. In fact, this is another way that Carrie Fisher was special in her stigma-busting: She made it clear that mental illness wasn't something that she had heroically conquered. She was wholeheartedly open about the complicated, chaotic, ongoing challenges of living with serious mental illness.

But, as with all the other anti-stigma approaches, demonstrating any longer-term impacts of this strategy beyond the news commentary seems difficult. Even more, there are plenty of examples of how celebrity advocacy can go wrong. US television host Katie Couric lost her husband to colon cancer in 1998. Two years later, she televised her own colonoscopy to destigmatize colon cancer screening. Screening rates went up—at least for a while—but mammography rates went down. It seems that many women who saw the experiment substituted a colonoscopy for a mammogram.[49] Studies have also shown how advocacy on behalf of stigmatized groups can also lead to serious blowback.[50] In 2016, the actress Amber Heard spoke out about the shaming and stigma she experienced after publically identifying as a victim of domestic violence. She was pilloried in the press as a liar and con artist.

Be an Activist

Some good successes have come from using activism to directly challenge stigmatizing beliefs and behaviors. Using a range of tactics—from petitions to boycotts to lawsuits to protests and civil disobedience—activism aims to disrupt (and even dismantle) existing social and power structures. Effective activism often comes directly from the grassroots mobilization of "communities of suffering," people with firsthand experiences of an illness who come together to encourage treatment and advance justice.[51] Such activism can sometimes challenge the structural causes of stigma in ways that have a significant impact.

SANE Australia, a mental health charity, devised a "stigma watch" program to help such communities fighting against mental illness stigma and to challenge damaging media depictions. Any member of the community that saw a stigmatizing portrayal could sound the alarm. SANE would then send a formal letter to media outlets or businesses explaining the complaint and suggesting fixes or removing the item. Many of the recipients seemed embarrassed by the callout and complied. SANE suggests this has made a real difference to how schizophrenia is portrayed in Australian media.[52] The power of such groups to create positive change through activism depends on many factors, including how much political savvy and media access the group can harness. SANE Australia, for example, has a board and patronage populated with doctors, professors, lawyers, and the former governor-general. Social class can make a big difference: Those with money and connections seem to be able to push back the hardest.

A good example of the combined power of activism and high social status is the success of AIDS Coalition to Unleash Power (ACT UP) in the United States. In the 1980s, HIV/AIDS was a newly identified disease, perceived as a "gay plague" and carrying with it the promise of certain death. Overcoming fear, grief, and despair, gay HIV-positive men and their allies created a powerful social movement to fight the enormous stigma then attached to HIV/AIDS and LGBTQ+ status.[53] ACT UP and allied organizations used many forms of activism: protests, art and music, literature and press, scientific research and collaboration, and pressure on doctors and federal agencies.[54] Ultimately, they won stunning successes in scientific advancements, legislative victories, and shifts in public opinion. Today, the need for destigmatization is widely understood among global public health practitioners working on HIV/AIDS.[55] To understand the movement's success, it is important to acknowledge that ACT UP and other gay HIV-positive activists of the 1980s—while facing enormous homophobia and HIV/AIDS stigma—were disproportionately male, white, middle or upper class, and well-educated.[56] Higher social status helped the activists increase the impact of their activism in the realms of science, art, and media. In contrast, many communities of suffering have very few social privileges they can leverage in support of their activism.

Turning back to mental health, the overall *scientific* evidence on activism as an approach to addressing mental health stigma is equivocal as there have been very few actual studies. Diseases that are well-established, incurable, and widely associated with marginalized populations are less likely to see major, successful destigmatization campaigns. Once a disease "settles into" an association with poverty, much of the capacity to push back against stigma through activism and protest dissipates.[57] It becomes less of a media interest and less of a political concern.[58] Protests and other calls to action by those communities of suffering that are already disempowered, unpopular, or mistrusted may even then serve to bolster negative views about the disease.

Doing It All: Comprehensive Public Campaigns

Most large-scale campaigns today try to use a broad anti-stigma tool kit to relabel, reeducate, reframe, connect, leverage celebrity advocates, and work in collaboration with local activists all at once. Does this multi-pronged approach lead to better outcomes? The World Psychiatric Association launched the "Open the Doors" (OTD) global anti-stigma campaign in 1996.[59] They chose to focus on schizophrenia as the most widely feared and one of the most serious mental illnesses. The stated aim of the OTD was "to dispel the myths and misunderstandings."[60] The goal was for people with schizophrenia to be able to work, go to school, be with their families, and live with hope. To date some twenty-one countries from Austria to Uganda have rolled out OTD programming.[61]

OTD was important because it was the first long-term, large-scale, anti-stigma effort, rolled out across multiple countries and sustained through time. It required in-depth partnering with multiple local organizations. Strategies varied from place to place but included social marketing to increase public knowledge and shift perceptions of the disease being untreatable. The campaigns used websites, television ads, public lectures, and art exhibits to get the message out. They held community social events to connect people. They supported activists, pushing governments for greater spending on mental health services or improved legal protections around discrimination. Local celebrities were deployed to spread the word.

Sadly, it seems that OTD was not nearly as successful as was hoped, given the level of investment and effort. But it is hard to say with any certainty because there was no emphasis in the OTD (or other similar campaigns) on systematically tracking the resulting changes in how people think and behave.[62] Say, for example, the goal is to reduce stigma so that people with mental illness find it less challenging to rent housing. These types of concrete outcomes were simply not monitored.[63]

Still, overall, the evidence suggests that even fully coordinated de-stigmatization efforts in high-income countries mostly fail, especially when they are trying to change attitudes around severe or "settled in" illnesses like schizophrenia.[64] Since serious action to challenge mental illness stigma started a half-century ago, public stigma has barely changed at all, and yet the strategies employed have also largely remained the same.[65]

Moreover, this largely ineffective approach is now being exported from high-income to low-income nations.[66] The World Health Organization's stance is that, "Public education and awareness campaigns on mental health should be launched in all countries."[67] Norman Satorius, the Croatian psychiatrist who ran the World Health Organization mental health program from 1967–1993, led the development of OTD. He has long been committed to the idea that global mental health can only improve if we first handle stigma.[68] He also has been open in discussing the flaws in the WHO anti-stigma efforts. His basic conclusion was that "stigma should be tackled in a fundamentally different way from most of the efforts carried out so far."

We agree. Launching copycat campaigns in low- and middle-income countries is a fundamentally flawed idea. We suspect they will cost a bundle and do very little.[69] Worse, they could do real damage. Each mental health anti-stigma effort will need to be highly tailored, and in sophisticated ways, to each and every place they are delivered. Then the impacts need to be followed carefully to reduce unwanted blowback effects or other unintended damage. (The good news is that relatively simplistic and low-cost social media monitoring can produce a rough longitudinal estimate of stigma shifts at a country-wide level.) This matters even more for low-income countries with high inequality—given that resources are limited and the power differences between the public health and medical establishment and the people being treated can be substantial.

Consider one of the simplest and most straightforward strategies, the local relabeling of serious illnesses like bipolar disorder or epilepsy to reduce stigma. Without the necessary ethnographic and linguistic groundwork to discern the cultural and moral roots of how and why the illnesses are stigmatized in that specific context, there is a pretty good chance efforts will go belly-up.[70] And if you don't bother to track shifts in stigma afterward, you won't even know this has happened.

Mental illness can be debilitating and needs medical treatment, and stigma can easily interfere with this. This leads to a fundamental question that no one seems to be asking: In the wake of all this repeated effort and failure, is full removal of the stigma from severe mental illness even *possible*? We address this question next by investigating whether there are any societies where the stigma of mental illness is adequately managed.

The Bottom Line

Profound stigma means those struggling with mental illness can endure lives of rejection, treated as unwanted and useless. This worsens mental illness treatment at every turn. Recognizing this, destigmatization has been a core strategy in mental health efforts for half a century. Most current efforts are aimed at removing public stigma. Public health is doing a poor job of tracking how stigma changes and how this impacts the daily lives of people diagnosed with mental illness. Our best guess: It mostly fails.

The Myth of the Destigmatized Society

In the 1990s, the World Health Organization (WHO) published what has been described as the most important findings ever in psychiatric epidemiology,[1] the International Study of Schizophrenia (ISoS).[2] The study was based on epidemiological data collected for 1,704 people in seventeen sites over the course of fifteen years, including India, Colombia, Ireland, and the Czech Republic. The study began by identifying a subset of those people in different countries who had contacted psychiatric services, examined them using a standard protocol for core symptoms of schizophrenia, then track what happened to them for at least two years afterward. One of the study's aims was to see if there were differences between lower- and higher-income countries and how people with schizophrenia fared over time after they were diagnosed.

The study leads concluded that people diagnosed with schizophrenia in low- and middle-income countries (LMIC) did better, over time, than those in high-income countries (HIC). They were less likely to display signs of schizophrenia after treatment, were less reliant on antipsychotic medication once released from hospital and appeared to be better integrated into their communities.[3] At several sites, there was an extraordinary finding: The *majority* of those diagnosed with schizophrenia were free of symptoms years later. For example, of the cohort of one hundred patients followed in Chennai, India, only eight had shown continuous signs of illness five years later. This wasn't to say everyone in low-income countries got better, but their odds of doing so appeared significantly higher.[4] They were also more likely to be "working." This was considered extraordinarily good news about a potentially debilitating, chronic—and some even argue incurable—disease. The Geneva-based director of WHO's Department of Mental Health said at the time, "If I become psychotic, I'd rather be in India than in Switzerland."[5]

These findings were especially surprising given that people in LMIC have much poorer access to mental health treatment. For example, the WHO's own Global Health Observatory shows that there is one psychiatrist for every 7,000 or so residents in the Western European countries that reported data. In India, there is one psychiatrist per 330,000 residents. In some of the poorest countries in Africa, it is one per 10 million. Why would India—with its lack of doctors, drugs, and all other health resources that should matter—have such better outcomes than Switzerland, sometimes said to have one of the best health-care systems in the world? Cultural differences, particularly tied to the stigma of mental illness, were used to explain these widely varying outcomes for people diagnosed with schizophrenia. But determining exactly how stigma might matter for long-term outcomes depends on how you organize and interpret the evidence. Two very different stories can be told.

Story A: Smaller-Scale Societies Promote Less Suffering

The first version of the story was the one often told by the WHO study leaders. They concluded that recovery was better in LMIC because those with schizophrenia had less complex social demands placed on them and more family support.[6] This was embedded in the greater cultural acceptance of people with mental illnesses. Not having to struggle with rejection, hostility, and mistreatment in their daily lives, people recovered faster from illness episodes and did better over time.

In this story, the underlying reason for better outcomes is that many people in LMIC live in communities and families where relationships come first. In these *sociocentric* societies, people place priority on sustaining long-term relationships. Collective family and community needs are more important than individual desires. In such settings, support is expected at some level for all members, even those with severe challenges. As a result, people with signs of schizophrenia are less likely to be rejected, isolated, or institutionalized (figure 8.1).[7] Instead, they get love and caring from family and friends.

Studies of people with schizophrenia from Japan, Hong Kong, and Singapore—highly industrialized societies but with family-oriented cultures—seem to support this theory. Extended kin networks provide social connections, better tolerate "strange" symptoms, and generally buffer against stigma.[8] By contrast, the nuclear family rules in places like the United States and United Kingdom, and people have few real, formalized obligations to cousins, distant aunts, or other extended family. They only need to help if they want to. This means people who are sick are more likely to be pushed toward hospital treatment and other forms of institutional care.

Some cross-cultural studies from smaller-scale societies have helped bolster this story version. In 1970, sociologist Nancy Waxler followed people diagnosed with schizophrenia (PDWS) after they were discharged from a Sri Lankan psychiatric ward in 1970. She then tracked them down five years later to see how they were doing.[9] The PDWS were mostly Buddhist farmers, so had modest means and lifestyle. The large, strong Sinhalese families were highly tolerant of their family members' differences and limitations. They willingly took them back into their homes after treatment and accepted the extra work to care for them. Family members described schizophrenia as troublesome but curable. They said this often and in the presence of those affected, and they didn't blame the person for their illness. For Waxler, this absence of stigma was what drove excellent long-term outcomes for PDWS, including the low rate of hospital readmission.

The Sinhalese view of the curability of schizophrenia contrasts sharply with the perceptions of schizophrenic relapse that continue to dominate in high-income nations and that reinforce the condition's inevitable chronicity—that the disease would persist and that full

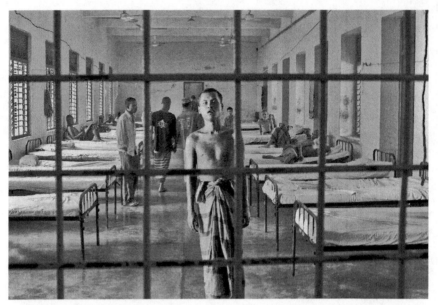

Figure 8.1. A patient looks through the windows of Pabna Mental Hospital, the first and oldest mental hospital in Bangladesh, founded in 1957. © 2011 Fahad Bin Solaiman, courtesy of Photoshare

recovery was mostly hopeless. American families from a wide array of backgrounds, for example, are more hostile toward family members with schizophrenia because they see the condition as unrecoverable. In turn, this makes them less willing to care for the relative at home. Medical institutions must take over, and, as Erving Goffman had explained, they then make people even crazier.[10]

Importantly, Waxler's Sri Lankan study suggested that the destigmatization of severe mental illness is a real possibility. It also provided some clues about the best way to do it: teach the hope of recovery. It provided an early, optimistic view of what could be possible. The broader view of the crucial role of cultural factors play in success for treating schizophrenia also highlights that interventions should be focused in the community and how people are treated as patients, neighbors, and family members.[11]

Story B: Smaller-Scale Societies Promote More Suffering

The other interpretation of the complex cross-national evidence around schizophrenia is a less hopeful one. Story B challenges the WHO conclusions that small-scale societies in low- and middle-income countries are somehow safe spaces for people with mental illness, rather suggesting that people diagnosed with schizophrenia in LMIC may suffer more, not less. Part of the argument against the WHO conclusions is based on criticism of the study design itself.[12] For one thing, the finding representing all "developing" countries was based in data for only 234 people from India and 138 from Colombia. And moreover, the study recruited people who were admitted to hospitals: Hospital treatment for mental illness is less available to those in low-income countries to begin with. Families hiding away sick members to avoid shame would be less likely to show up at a hospital regardless. Two participants in one study of PDWS in India were beaten to death when wandering at night.[13] Dead people also don't show up as hospital admissions.

But, also, Story A doesn't fit well with what anthropologists tend to observe on the ground. For one thing, the classic signs of schizophrenia—with its myriad emotional and social miscues—are interpreted as "odd," "wrong," or "off" in all kinds of societies. As early as the mid-1970s, cultural anthropologist Jane Murphy wrote about this phenomenon in her ethnographic work with Yupik-speaking people in the Bering Sea and the Egba Yoruba in Nigeria.[14] At the time, no one in either place had any concept of schizophrenia as a disease. But when they saw people exhibiting the signs of schizophrenia, they knew something wasn't quite right, like a sickness in desperate need of a cure.

Our colleague, biological anthropologist Karen Schmidt, has studied people's reactions to the signs of severe mental illness in two very different settings: New Zealand Māori in Auckland and Papua New Guineans in Port Moresby.[15] She interviewed PDWS on video, asking them to answer questions like: What was it like growing up in (your country)? Where do you think your country is headed in the future? Can you tell me a little about yourself?

Schmidt then asked members of the public to watch and rate the videos from both sites. The facial cues were enough for viewers to easily identify the people diagnosed with schizophrenia as "odd," even if they didn't understand the language they were speaking. People diagnosed with schizophrenia tend to have a hard time emoting in the same way others do, and one common sign is that they display "fake" smiles. These seem unspontaneous because it takes too long for the corners of the mouth to elevate.[16] The viewers didn't understand what they were seeing, but they *knew* that something wasn't quite right.

It appears that the "that's not right" reactions to the signs of schizophrenia and other severe mental illnesses occur in all human societies. Sociologist Bernice Pescosolido and her colleagues told the following story to people in sixteen different countries:[17]

> Up until a year ago, life was pretty okay for John. But then, things started to change. He thought that people around him were making disapproving comments and talking behind his back. John was convinced that people were spying on him and that they could hear what he was thinking. John lost his drive to participate in his usual work and family activities and retreated to his home, eventually spending most of his time on his own. John became so preoccupied with what he was thinking that he skipped meals and stopped bathing regularly. At night, when everyone else was sleeping, he was walking back and forth at home. John was hearing voices even though no one else was around. These voices told him what to do and what to think. He has been living this way for six months.

The researchers found that in a wide array of places, even where schizophrenia wasn't well-known as a concept, people responded similarly to the vignette. They didn't want John to be around children, feared he would be unpredictable and violent, and didn't want him to marry into their family.

Why do the signs of oddness associated with mental illness cause us to want social distance so consistently? It may be hardwired into our brains, part of being a species that relies so heavily on social interaction for survival. Moreover, there is an ever-growing set of ethnographic studies that suggest people with symptoms of severe mental illness are poorly treated in small- and large-scale societies alike.[18] If you look carefully, rejection, shunning, mocking, and abuse of people with signs of mental illness are found everywhere—even in India, one of the key sites of the WHO study.

In the interviews done by public health scholar Kaaren Mathias in Western Utter Pradesh in northern India, we can see an example of this. Raju, a middle-aged man with schizophrenia, explained his experiences of mental illness and stigma. He told researchers, "Not just outsiders but my family also maintained distance . . . even my wife and children. I feel bad still as my children do not talk to me. I feel hurt when my children do not come to me often."

Nilofer, the same age and from the same village said, "My husband does not tell me when he takes some decision. When I ask him something, he says 'Why do you need to know? You are mad' . . . And my sisters-in-law didn't even allow me to bathe in their bathrooms. After my child was born, I had to raise the cot on all sides and take my bath there . . . And then, when they let me use their bathroom just occasionally, they would wash their bathroom afterward, as if I had some bad disease. I felt really bad at that time.

Their neighbor, 35-year-old Faiz, said similar things about her middle-aged brother: "No friend of his has ever come to see him. When he goes out, he recognizes people, but people do not talk to him. People say he is mad and there is no use talking to him . . . No one actually hates my brother, but I wish that people would stop pitying him. People keep saying, "Poor fellow, what has become of him?" But no one says anything to him at all, and instead they talk about him amongst themselves."[19]

One of the most convincing studies that supports Story B was based in rural villages to the south of Chengdu, China. House-by-house interviews revealed 510 adults who had exhibited signs of schizophrenia then or in the past.[20] Two years later, a third of these patients had received no medical treatment. Mostly this was due to a lack of money and relatives deciding that professional help was unnecessary. Those patients who had stayed solely in the care of families were doing much worse; most had obvious symptoms like delusions of persecution or severe social withdrawal. Other studies in places such as India and Ethiopia have shown similar results. Even in the most rural, family-centered societies, people not being treated for schizophrenia tend to have more symptoms and more related disability. Once they are taken from homecare and placed into medical treatment, they tend to do significantly better.

What Helps Most

This is a key point in weighing Story A and Story B: It isn't just industrialized societies that make serious social demands on people, small-scale societies can too. A large extended family might give you support when you are sick and needy, but they also make demands on you in return. You may be expected to hold down a job and contribute money to support them, organize complex funereal rites when they die, or help find good spouses to help care for them and their children. These are exactly the types of complex, stressful social obligations that people with severe mental illness often struggle with the most.[21]

One revealing finding from the Chengdu, China, study is that three-quarters of those untreated were still managing to work at least part-time two years later. In this rural area, some form of valued productivity was still possible even for those with severe symptoms. Women could still often perform the expected combination of household tasks, childcare, and farming. However, this doesn't mean these village societies are less stigmatizing. It does mean that there are socially acceptable, productive roles available that can accommodate some of the symptoms of mental illness, even though the symptoms are still viewed as highly undesirable.

Ethnographic studies can help us better understand what is going on here, and why it matters for managing mental illness stigma. Anthropologist Roger Sullivan spent several seasons in Palau working with psychiatrists and patients at Belau National Hospital.[22] A small Micronesian island-nation in the Pacific Ocean east of the Philippines, Palau has the highest reported rates of schizophrenia in the world. The rates are unusually high for men, almost twice that of women, which is surprising given that most studies show women are considerably more at risk of diagnosis.

Sullivan has been trying to unravel why men are more at risk than women in Palau to determine if demanding social roles are to blame. He found that the clinical symptoms of the disease here looked generally the same as elsewhere, and certainly negatively affected people's lives. Like some of the LMIC in the original WHO ten-country study, Palau treats the majority of people with diagnosed schizophrenia, especially those with milder cases, as outpatients. Most live at home with their families. But a major and important difference is that Palauan women diagnosed with schizophrenia were more likely to get married and have children than Palauan men.

In Palauan culture, the social and economic "value" assigned to women is generally higher than that assigned to men (figure 8.2).[23] Traditional Palauan society is strictly matrilineal, which means that land, titles, and inheritance are passed down through women. Men's social standing and marriageability relies on their capacity to hold down a job and earn in the cash economy. Women, on the other hand, are viewed as "earners" even if they don't work outside the home, because when they marry, have children, or even when they divorce, the husband's family will pay cash for goods (such as a new house). Accordingly, families are motivated to support adult women even when the going gets tough. The prognosis for women with schizophrenia, who can still provide a valued social role, is much better than for men with the disease, who may find it difficult to hold down a paying job and, therefore, have no social standing.

This example shows that what seems to matter most is the capacity of the person to adjust to fit morally and socially acceptable roles and niches. In Palau, women with symptoms of schizophrenia are still able to marry and have children. That means they can be successful in achieving the cherished family goals of creating new kinship and inheritance. As a result, it's more possible for women's families (and society at large) to deny, ignore, or tolerate stigmatized symptoms and diagnoses. The stigma is there, but the social dysfunction isn't— or at least not so much that it matters.

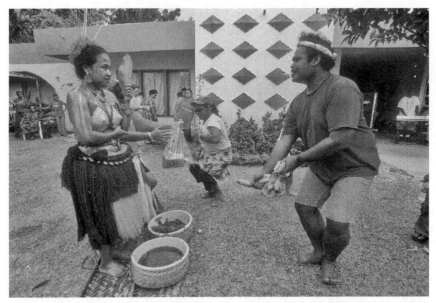

Figure 8.2. A young mother is presented with gifts by her husband's family after the birth of her first child, Palau, Micronesia, 2005. © Alamy

Ethnographically informed studies like this one in Micronesia provide the needed clarity about why culture matters in stigma studies. Social demands, shaped by norms about what is culturally expected to be "successful," can make or break people. When people can't find a way to contribute in ways that are locally valued, they suffer. But when people can meet cultural expectations, they take on social roles and identities that are positive enough to balance out their devalued, stigmatized ones. Mathematician John Nash, whose life was portrayed in the award-winning film *A Beautiful Mind*, lived with obvious signs of schizophrenia but was also seen as a genius. The latter identity allowed him to work on and off in Ivy League academic jobs through decades of serious illness, culminating in the receipt of the 1994 Nobel Prize in Economics.

Similarly, stigma can be lessened when people have other, more valued social roles, even when those roles come, ironically, from having a stigmatized condition. Take, for example, a case of people living in extreme poverty in New York City.[24] Being labeled as mentally ill is highly stigmatizing. But if people are placed by their doctors on long-term disability because of their mental illness, psychiatric outpatients earn a relatively steady (if small) income. This income can help support a family and provide stable housing. As such, it can generate the forms of respect especially important to men faced with the social requirement that they act as breadwinners—as we see very clearly in the tragic story of Kumar and his Nepalese family in the next chapter. Women are more often able to manage the stay-at-home status with less innate stigma than men. This gendered access to social roles that allow valued forms of productivity while managing mental illness can explain in part why outcomes can be different for men and women.

Engineering Social Roles?

When it comes to mental illness, social roles are very important for determining if stigma becomes utterly incapacitating or more of a nuisance. Stigma's effect can be lessened by people's participation in socially valued roles. What helps is finding ways that people with severe mental illness can successfully inhabit socially valued roles—especially roles that offset the stigmatized identity. At that same time, it is important to remember that social demands that are too burdensome can be harmful to people with delicate mental health.

If social roles matter most, then we need a completely new agenda for how to deal with destigmatization in mental illness. This means abandoning the long-term emphasis on public education that has been favored in the past. Instead, we need to be identifying and creating social roles in which people with mental illnesses can contribute to and participate in society and the economy. This suggests that our approaches should be systematic, but culturally informed and culturally specific. What works for men may not work for women; what works for farmers may not work for urbanites. We need to look closely at social roles and find places where people with stigmatized conditions can succeed in them. And it suggests that all the effort to change public opinions about stigmatized mental illness may be a costly distraction from the more complex, important work that needs to be done.

To complicate things further, the definition of what are accessible and acceptable social roles is in flux right now. Gender roles are changing in many places, with stay-at-home dads and working moms gaining greater social acceptability. With globalization, there is a move away from farming and other subsistence lifestyles. The new demands of the cash economy—holding down a job, completing a degree, or being successful in a highly competitive dating and marriage market—are based much more on looks.[25] In many ways, it becomes increasingly difficult to find the types of jobs that can easily accommodate people who deviate from the prevailing norms of acceptable appearance and behavior.[26]

We can expect things to change even more in coming years. Efforts to "disrupt" industries using computer and robotic technology are expected to decrease employment globally. Tech titans have begun discussing whether universal basic income, a living stipend for everyone, might be a way to deal with this potential rise in underemployment and unemployment. This thought experiment gives us the opportunity to rethink the socioeconomic organization of our society. Are there ways we can redesign our working lives so that everyone can be socially valued, so everyone can contribute meaningfully? This is an important question, and one we return to in the next chapter as we consider how notions of being useless and unproductive—of having no value in society—don't just stem from mental illness but can also drive them.

The Bottom Line

Stigma toward severe mental illness is evident even in small-scale, family-focused societies. This suggests that, while stigma can be reduced, it might never be removed. But the ethnographic record also shows that help with fitting in through access to valued social roles can help significantly with reducing dysfunction and improve long-term prognosis.

Completely Depressing

Our colleague Ashley Hagaman recently completed eighteen months of field research in mountainous Nepal.[1] She has been investigating the social triggers of suicide in this small, South Asian, mainly Hindu, nation. Her time was split between noisy, bustling Kathmandu and the quiet, snow-capped rural district of Jumla. Suicide rates in urban and rural Nepal are estimated to be some of the highest in the world,[2] although suicide is widely underreported. Part of the problem is that suicide is both illegal and highly stigmatized.

To get around suicide underreporting, Hagaman used a "psychological autopsy" approach to find cases of suicide that were not reported. Hagaman scoured police and hospital records, and when she found a potential case of suicide, she tracked down more information by talking to others in the local community. Finally, she would approach the family and close friends. Many were willing to share painful stories about what might have led the person to die by suicide (figure 9.1).

One of the cases Hagaman tracked was a young man named Kumar. Like many Nepalese men, Kumar's social standing (*ijat*) was important to him and depended on his ability to be a good financial provider. In talking about his death, his relatives told stories about a disastrous work trip he took to Malaysia.

Kumar had arranged to take a high-earning job at a prestigious hotel in Malaysia. The family invested their life savings into paying

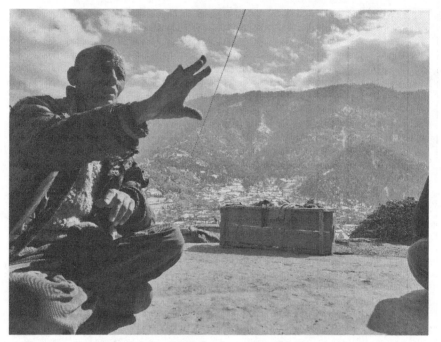

Figure 9.1. As part of a verbal autopsy, a family member discusses the circumstances of suicide, Nepal. Photo by A. Hagaman

the up-front costs—immigration fees, bribes, a middle man—so Kumar could work abroad in Malaysia and send money home to Nepal. When he arrived in Malaysia, the promised prestigious hotel job turned out to be a scam.

Kumar found himself hauling heavy furniture parts in an unbearably hot factory. He was forced to work more than twelve hours each day without adequate breaks. He fell ill. He desperately wanted to return to Nepal, and he begged his family for help. It was two months before they could pull together enough cash to get him out of the labor contract and onto a plane.

His uncle explained what happened next:

When he came back from Malaysia, he felt ashamed because he could not bring any money or anything. He couldn't do anything for his family, you know? He came back with nothing. There were also so many problems with his wife . . . she couldn't take it anymore, so she left. They said it was because he couldn't earn money and that he was foolish. Everyone [else] told him it was his fault. All these things, they destroyed his *ijat*. They destroyed him.

Despite his family's efforts to make him feel better, Kumar was wracked with guilt. He knew he was now a burden. He wasn't the man he should be. The loss of his *ijat* brought shame to his family, who he knew deserved better. Kumar killed himself by hanging at the age of twenty-two. The note he left to his wife simply said, "You left me. My life is meaningless. I won't able to live in this place, so now I am leaving."

Many other stories Hagaman collected explained suicide in this way: a failure to live up to other people's expectations for how you *should* be. In Nepal, loss of *ijat* is so laden with dreadful meaning that it drives people to take their own lives.[3] Certainly, as we explored in chapter 7, stigma seriously inhibits people's recovery from mental illness. And so, even if most destigmatization efforts fail, we must keep trying to find better solutions that work.

The story of Kumar and millions other like him speaks to how stigma unravels our core sense of self and washes away the meaning of our existence. How stigma drives forward our mental illness, such as depression and even suicide, is the focus of this chapter.

Social Disadvantage and Depression

We have been studying for several years how stigmatized social failures so easily shape unipolar depression. Feeling sad, tired, and hopeless sometimes are inherent parts of being human. It is normal for us to feel grief when someone we love dies or to be despondent when we are rejected for a job we really want. However, depression occurs when the low mood persists for an extended period, and it is often accompanied by disabling self-criticism, apathy, fatigue, and social withdrawal. It may even manifest itself as physical aches and pain. Depression often co-occurs with anxiety and is a major contributing factor to suicide.[4]

In milder cases, people can often muddle through their daily lives, albeit with feelings of inadequacy and fatigue. With severe depression, though, it is hard to do even basic tasks. You struggle to get out of bed, let alone to meet the demands of work, raising a family, and functioning as part of a community. Even the most basic social interaction—the interpersonal give-and-take of daily living—can be excruciating.

Depression thrives in adversity. Rates skyrocket whenever there is conflict, hunger, chronic physical illness, or massive social and economic inequality. It is, therefore, no surprise that India—a country with extreme poverty, social inequality, and a history of famine and natural disasters—is among the most depressed and anxious nations in the world. Around a third of the Indian population is thought to have suffered at least one major depressive episode at some stage in their lives.[5] Countries with even worse socioeconomic conditions (for example, those in the wake of civil war, famine, or humanitarian disaster) contain even greater numbers of people with anxiety or depression. For example, Liberia in West Africa, which endured a traumatizing five-year civil war in the early 2000s, had depression rates of about 40 percent for years to follow.[6]

But it doesn't take war, disaster, or extreme poverty to increase the incidence of depression. Seemingly small, everyday social rejections and micro-stigmatizations are also building blocks for depression. In rural Uganda, where rates of HIV and AIDS are extremely high, almost a quarter of adults are depressed at any time. The high depression rates are attributed partly to poverty and partly to illness-related stressors. However, the major factor in driving depression appears to be the stigma associated with HIV/AIDS.[7]

Depression also increases in groups fighting their own daily battles against inequality and social exclusion. For example, in the United States, members of racially minoritized groups experience casual, everyday degradations ("microaggressions"), or subtle (and often unintentional) discriminatory treatment. Asking someone, "Why don't you have an accent?" or saying, "But you look so white!"

are subtle, but pernicious, forms of racism. They predict higher levels of blood pressure, depression, and other clinical correlates of stress.[8]

Gender discrimination causes similar damaging stress. For example, in rural northern Pakistan, women have little opportunity to become literate and educated. They have little chance to gain formal employment or own property or goods. Rural women in northern Pakistan must cede to male authority in many areas of their lives. They struggle with poverty. This reflects prevailing, established social norms and the way institutions are designed to run in Pakistan. But living as second-class citizens, alongside their more powerful husbands and fathers, causes as many as half of Pakistani women to suffer from depression or anxiety, or both.[9]

These connections between stigma, women's disempowerment, and depression were apparent in our study of Uzbek women living in the wake of national independence.[10] Under Soviet rule, the law required that women have access to education and employment. The removal of Soviet power in Uzbekistan in the 1990s led to a resurgence in certain Islamic traditions that subjugated women. As a result, women were removed from schools, pushed out of jobs, and many were no longer permitted to go to the doctor or shop alone. We identified high rates of depression among women overall, much higher than among men. Moreover, the very highest rates were among women who *believed* they should have real autonomy. Women who were fine with the new social order—who didn't think it was patently unfair—had relatively better mental health.

Food, Social Failure, and Depression

Anthropologist Lesley Jo Weaver has been doing fieldwork in Brazil recently to study the links between food and depression.[11] Like the United States, Brazil is a huge, diverse country with many social and economic inequalities. People are discriminated against and socially discredited based on many factors. For example, not having a slim body shape, not having light skin, and not eating the right high-prestige foods (like pizza and ice cream)[12] all mark you as being "behind the times," "unmodern," and less important to an advancing country. Weaver interviewed men and women living in six hundred households in a farming community, where the standard cuisine is rice, beans, and meat. For them, a shameful diet lacked variety, contained little meat, and wasn't cooked fresh. At the same time, most people didn't think food insecurity was a problem, because as far as they could tell their neighbors always had enough to share. Herein lies the rub.

Certainly, being short of food is depressing. Weaver, along with our colleague Craig Hadley, has shown that experiences of food insecurity make people more likely to suffer anxiety and depression all over the world.[13] But the deep shame of not having enough food to meet social expectations is what seems to really intensify depression. The more people understand they are failing socially, and struggle to meet those norms, the more depressed they seem to become. Food is something we must deal with every day of our lives. It is also at the core of how we relate to others in our family and our community, by sharing meals. Food sits at the heart of our social relationships.

Similar to *ijat* in Nepal, it isn't the shortage of food alone that depresses people. It is about a failure to live up to basic social expectations. Giving and receiving food is a key social activity in the Brazilian community where Weaver conducted research. You should offer a plate of food to neighbors after an event or invite friends who stop by to join your table. Weaver explains that the shame and self-stigma of not having enough food makes people desperate to hide their food shortages from others. As a result, they can't engage in food reciprocity, nor explain why they are defaulting.

Luisa, who lived on the edge of the community, explained it by saying, "We do what we can. Sometimes we have to eat only rice with nothing on top of it. That's it. That's how it is for us. We don't have to be ashamed of how our situation is, it is normal." Luisa's statement of "We don't have to be ashamed," ironically shows just how humiliating it really is for her. The shame of food insecurity, as much as food insecurity itself, was driving depressive symptoms in households like Luisa's. In addition, not having enough food to connect socially with neighbors was also socially isolating, which is another major risk factor for depression. But which families were the most depressed of all? The worst symptoms were experienced by those who were driven by shame to buy and share luxury food items that they simply couldn't afford.

These types of daily social failures are making people depressed in countries all over the world, not just in places like Nepal and Uzbekistan and Brazil, where globalization and social change are wreaking havoc. Arizona State University anthropologist Ben Trumble has been working with a large team of anthropologists to track health shifts among the Tsimané hunter-gatherers of lowland Bolivia. While Trumble's field site is in the same small country as Amber's, it would take her seven days of uncomfortable travel by bus, canoe, and foot to get from her field site in Cochabamba to the Tsimané villages where Ben works.

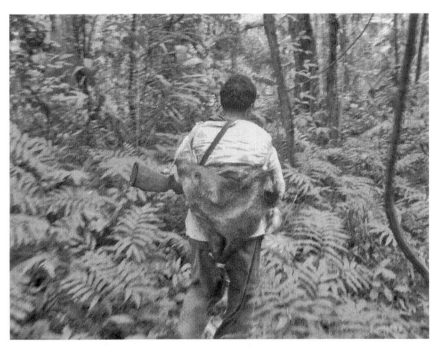

Figure 9.2. Tsimané hunter bringing home a peccary, Bolivia. Photo by B. Trumble

The Tsimané are rainforest hunters and swidden farmers. They earn a little additional cash by selling wood or farming bananas and manioc, or taking small jobs at the market town of San Borja. They live in about ninety highly social, family-based villages. The Tsimané have a relatively fair, egalitarian society where both men and women can have a voice of authority. Elders are heeded, and older people look after younger. People are *expected* to share. They are *expected* to support each other.

The Tsimané understand depression and can feel it intensely.[14] They describe it as *yoquedye'* ("thinking too much"), which doesn't exactly match the English description.[15] To them, depression is worry, pure and simple; it is about losing someone you love or the effects of a serious illness. But what makes people most distressed? When Trumble's team surveyed the Tsimané, in asking what they would change in their lives to be happier, bringing home more food and sharing it more with others topped the list. The least productive adults were the most depressed, because they felt they were failing to meet their obligations and worried about getting their families enough to eat. Moreover, because the older Tsimané are expected to be better hunters and fisherfolk and thus provide more, being both older and unproductive proved the most depressing combination of all (figure 9.2).[16]

Across societies, depression symptoms generally correlate with people's deep concerns of who they *should be* in their daily lives. They also tell us a substantial amount about "what matters most" to people.[17] We seem to be especially likely to get depressed when we *feel we are utterly failing* to meet those expectations—when we know that others see our failings.[18] Nothing more clearly represents utter social failure than stigmatization, and any type of stigma can trigger depression—even very simple, almost incidental things like where you live.

The Depressing Stain of Tainted Places

Just down the road from our offices at Arizona State University is South Phoenix. We have been doing applied, community-based ethnographic research there since 2006, mostly around the issue of obesity.

Over the years, we had heard many people talk with pride and care about their community. They expressed positivity, appreciation, solidarity, and hope about living there. But people living outside of South Phoenix didn't tend to share this view, and it seems they never have.

The city of Phoenix emerged as a new, booming agricultural center in the late 1860s, on the remains of the abandoned ancient Hohokam canal system that distributed water from the Salt River. When the railway came through Phoenix in 1887, migrants arrived in search of work. Mostly Spanish-speaking, they were forced to live on the south side of the tracks. Their shacks and tents were clustered amid the stinking mills, factories, stockyards, and foundries that supported the growing city. Their homes in South Phoenix were cordoned off from the rest of the citizenry.

Reliable water, sewage, and paved roads were investments made only to the north of the tracks, where new, white-only neighborhoods like Scottsdale were rapidly expanding. By the start of World War II, only 5 percent of homes in South Phoenix met acceptable housing standards such as running hot and cold water and a flush toilet. With severe overcrowding and rampant poverty and malnutrition, newspapers reported that babies were dying at alarming rates, many from typhoid and tuberculosis.

From early on, those living in South Phoenix were clearly marked by the rest of the city as classic "unsanitary subjects."[19] Our colleague Bob Bolin has been studying the history of such injustice in these neighborhoods.[20] Bolin showed us a very telling 1879 local newspaper clipping:

> [They] do their washing and cooking on the sidewalks, and all manner of filth is thrown into the ditches. They have no outhouses, and the stench arising from the numerous adobe holes is simply fearful . . . Some portions of our town surpass that of the Chinese quarters in San Francisco for filth and stench.

This sense of contamination reinforced the physical separation of the occupants and their neighborhoods from the rest of the city. They were stained by place, and the place was stained by them.

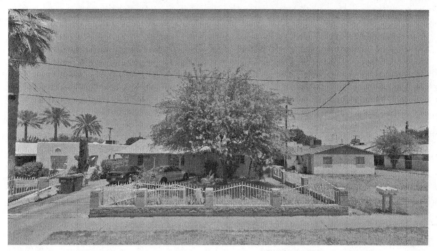

Figure 9.3. Residential street view in South Phoenix, Arizona, United States.

This stain has continued to be reflected in urban planning decisions made over the last century. The railways have shrunk in importance, but South Phoenix is now sandwiched between the mountains and downtown, two major freeways, and the main airport. The neighborhoods have dusty streets of small homes with pockets of factories and light industry (figure 9.3). Today, around two-thirds of South Phoenix's residents are Latinx and half of them were born outside the United States, mostly in Mexico.

We began to wonder: Lots of prior research has shown that living in poverty and health struggles can place people at risk of depression; could something as seemingly innocuous as feeling stigmatized for where you live also cause depression? This would be significant, given that previous studies had suggested the stigma of a place could stick with people long after they even lived there. One study showed that residents from public housing projects in Chicago remained tarred by their neighborhood's reputation for drugs and violence long after they had moved far away to Iowa.[21]

In 2013, we began to study the effects of neighborhood stigma by recruiting and interviewing eighty-four people in two Phoenix, Arizona, area neighborhoods: lower-income South Phoenix and nearby

North Scottsdale.[22] North Scottsdale is a place of prestige and comfort, often seen as a vacation delight with luxurious spas and cowboy kitsch, predominantly wealthy and almost 90 percent white.[23] It has high-end retail stores and restaurants, along with well-maintained parks, lakes, golf courses. It is as socially distant as you can get from South Phoenix's lower-income, high percentage migrant neighborhoods, even though it is less than ten miles from the edge of one to the other. We asked our participants describe both their own and the other neighborhood. Residents of the predominantly Latinx South Phoenix described Scottsdale and its residents as rich, clean, and expensive. Scottsdale residents described the people of South Phoenix and their neighborhoods as poor, dirty, and full of criminals. It was classic stigma of place.

We also then interviewed three hundred Latinx people living in other parts of the city as a comparison later that same year, from demographically similar neighborhoods but without South Phoenix's stigmatized reputation. We also asked people about their health, the types of other stressors they had in their everyday lives, and what they thought was good and bad about their neighborhoods—things like whether there were parks and walkable streets, their relationships with neighbors, and graffiti, trash, and crime. We then measured their level of depression.

Compared with Latinx people in other similar, but unstigmatized neighborhoods, those living in South Phoenix were much more likely to perceive themselves as judged negatively because of where they lived. Those living in South Phoenix (28 percent), in low-income tracts (26 percent), in predominantly Latinx tracts (34 percent), and Latinx people (25 percent) were more likely than the overall sample (4 percent) to report they had been discriminated against or been treated badly because they lived in their neighborhood. Even once we took such factors as income, being Latino, and having low incomes into account, we found that South Phoenix residents also had much higher risk of exhibiting symptoms of depression.[24]

The simple stigma of living in the "wrong" place was emotionally distressing and depressing for people. While there isn't a lot of research yet from other locations, we suspect the same pattern is re-peated in the many stigmatized places around the world.[25]

Gender, Stigma, and Mental Health

Women are estimated to have higher rates of depression and anxi-ety at any time and across their lifetimes, something like one-and-a-half to two times the risk that men do globally.[26] The causes of this gender difference are not solely or particularly biological, but rather depression shadows adversity and social suffering associated with being female. These can then interact with biological vulnerabilities to exaggerate risk. For example, globally, women are more likely to be living in poverty than men.[27] Women are also more often held to ac-count for failures in how they or their family looks or eats or acts, such as having hungry or unacceptably dirty children. Much of this judgment is created or amplified by lack of resources.

Consider women's experience of infertility in Egypt. A couple's in-fertility triggers more psychological distress in women than men. Women are more often blamed for the couple's infertility itself, even though something like half the time the medical issue may be with the husband. Married women's social worth lies more immedi-ately in meeting expectations of motherhood compared to her hus-band's. Divorce becomes more likely in a society where men can start over with a new wife and women can't—and a divorced wife has much reduced social and economic circumstances compared to her former husband. Relative wealth matters to the equation of women's suffering as well, because the capacity to fix infertility, such as through in-vitro fertilization, is totally dependent on the ability to pay.[28] Infer-tility might be something that happens to both the husband and the wife, but the blame and shame is far greater for women, and so too are its damaging psychological effects.

As we discussed earlier in the book regarding hygiene norms, gen-dered social standards for physical attractiveness tend to place dis-proportionate hygienic burdens on women and girls. In the wake of the Bangladeshi floods of 1998, the period of recovery was especially emotionally destructive for young, unmarried, menstruating women. There were much higher standards of modesty and cleanliness imposed on them, and they struggled to meet them every minute of every day. The ubiquitous floodwater made their clothing see-through and made them prone to harassment. Crowding meant they were at constant risk of being seen as they washed their menstrual cloths. Their sense of self-worth was replaced with constant worry and humiliation. One girl told of how she couldn't relax even when she was sleeping, because she was worried about someone seeing something they shouldn't. She lamented, "Can you imagine the *lajja* [shame] for us girls?"[29]

Women are also disproportionately exposed to domestic/intimate partner violence compared to men, which is, in itself, highly stigmatized. Globally at least one woman in three lives through serious physical abuse, such as a rape or severe beating.[30] Take the case of women sex workers living in the proximate cities of Beihai and Guilin, in Guangxi province, China.[31] The mostly young, minority women from nearby rural areas have little education or other skills to help them earn a living. Located near the Vietnamese border, these cities attract tourists willing and able to pay for sex. Around four thousand women work in the hair salons, karaoke bars, hotels, and massage parlors that front the trade. Their occupation is both illegal and highly stigmatized, yet it is an economic necessity for them and their families. They know they are judged as immoral, dirty, and diseased. They agree that they are shaming their families and themselves. However, what seems to do real and additional damage is not only the stigma of the sex work, but also the shame of intimate partner violence (IPV). Women are more likely to suffer verbal abuse, too. As one Serbian woman living with domestic violence explains, "Emotional abuse is worse. You can become insane when you are constantly humiliated and told that you are worthless, that you are nothing."[32] All this helps explain why being female adds to a potent cocktail for stigma-driven depression.[33] Being raped, kicked, slapped, dragged, humiliated, and belittled by a sexual partner is a major predictor of depression and suicidal thoughts.

Self-Reinforcing Stigma Cycles

We suspect highly damaging, self-reinforcing cycles of stigma and depression are causing millions to suffer all over the globe. But there has been almost no epidemiological work to show if and how this happens. One exception is a study of young children orphaned by HIV in Henan Province in central China, one of the poorest regions in the country.[34] Unfortunately, this study shows how awful such cycles can be.

In the late 1980s and early 1990s, impoverished rural Henan adults sold their blood at a poorly managed, government-run scheme. Having numerous donors hooked to the same blood-plasma machines led to a sudden and deadly epidemic of HIV. The count may have been as high as one million adults infected. Their children, too young to donate blood, were left behind as orphans. In the words of one of these 9-year-old girls,

> [After my parents died], the kids in the village did not play with me anymore. Nobody in school wants to speak with me. I have not spoken to anyone for a long time because no one will listen to me . . . I wanted to speak with my good friend before, but she is not willing to talk to me at all and always covers her mouth with her hand. Today, I finally found someone I can talk to: the big, yellow dog in my family. He is quietly listening when I talk and he will cry when I cry.[35]

Many thousands of these young children were rejected by their extended families. They ended up in the government-run orphanages set up to respond to the crisis. Most found that the physical living conditions were an improvement over the mud huts they left behind,[36] but they were socially tainted by their parents' stigmatized deaths. This stigma was reinforced because people were not only afraid of HIV; they also viewed giving blood as something only poor, desperate people did.

For three consecutive years, Henan children with HIV-infected parents and AIDS orphans were tracked, recording their awareness of stigma around HIV/AIDS, the level of mistreatment they felt from others, and their levels of depression. Children were asked if they were teased or picked on, ignored by relatives, or otherwise mistreated because of how their parents had died. What emerged was a portrait of a vicious cycle. Children who reported more mistreatment became more depressed. Depression seemed to make them more aware of and alert to their stigma and mistreatment. This then led to more stigmatized treatment by others, then more depression.

This is one of the few direct cases where the empirical effects of layered vulnerabilities have been unraveled and disassociated in a way that recognizes their additive, layered, intersecting, and compounding effects. In ethnographic fieldwork, though, we anecdotally observe this again and again, manifested as cycles of anger, frustration, depression, and illness. We need a lot more data-driven epidemiological studies to better help those trapped inside these awful cycles.

The Real Challenge: Compounded Stigma

Following Kimberlé Crenshaw's groundbreaking work[37] on intersectionality, social scientists have come to understand that axes of risks for stigma (such as being racially minoritized, female gendered, large-bodied, living in a devalued neighborhood, or belonging to a marginalized or disadvantaged social group) do not act alone. Black women in the United States, for example, experience multiple, overlapping, and compacting stigmas in ways that other stigma-sharers (e.g., white women and Black men) do not. Because Goffman's early work centered on dominant norms (implicitly understood to be male, white, heterosexual, etc.) and conceptualized stigma as a deviation from these norms,[38] the stigma literature has yet to fully address how intersectional experiences of stigma produce fundamentally different mental health risks.[39]

So, stigmas rarely travel solo. Disempowerment and isolation can hit from multiple angles: A person with untreated schizophrenia is also more likely to be unemployed, substance-using, homeless, and HIV positive. Each stigma then permits others by association. A poor person smoking crack is judged more harshly as a social failure and criminal than a rich one inhaling cocaine. People already living with the stigma of obesity are then judged more harshly for being unemployed or single, and so on.

Coping with stigma, depression, and social isolation can drive people to participate in risky, stigmatized behaviors like drug use, alcoholism, and stress eating. The depressive effects of stigma are, thus, often complexly compounded. One study in highly urban Baltimore, Maryland, USA, showed that homelessness is often a problem for heroin, crack, and cocaine users. Having no place to live caused depression, but this effect was small compared to the shame induced by their drug use. The compounding of shame-based depression made it harder to get off the streets, creating a downward spiral.[40]

Compounding this further, depressed people seem to be more aware that they are being stigmatized. Finally, the proverbial cherry on the cake: The more depressed you become, the more sensitive you are to feeling shamed and humiliated. In these ways, stigma and depression seem to feed off and intensify each other.

The power of stigma to depress and otherwise sicken in this way has been mostly invisible to public health and medicine to date. But there is good reason to suspect that stigma could be one of the basic drivers of global mental illness, as well as a fundamental and widespread cause of health inequalities.[41] Until we have contrary evidence, we need to act on the assumption that stigma is a major, mostly unrecognized global force, shaping and compounding depression and probably every other mental illness too.

The Bottom Line

Stigma strikes at the core of our social identities, telling us that we are devalued by others or should devalue ourselves. Multiple types of stigma and other forms of low power intersect, compounding people's distress. This worsens depression and other mental illness. Stigma is likely a major, unrecognized driver of global mental illness.

What We Can Do

Our goal in this book has been to show exactly how and why stigma creeps into public global health efforts, usually just outside of our vision, and the damage this does. We have also discussed how and why chronic, complex physical and mental health conditions—such as obesity, mental illness, and sanitation-related diseases—are extremely difficult to destigmatize. But there is much that *can* be done, and this is the focus of this final chapter. In fact, those who work in global public health are often best able to enact important changes in how we recognize and challenge stigma (figure C.1). Global health practice might be a source of some of the problems, but global health practitioners are themselves the keys to the solution.

How Do We Remove Stigma from Global Public Health Efforts?

Obviously perhaps, the most effective way to undo the damage of stigma within public health is to prevent it from happening in the first place. So, as a first, crucial, fundamental point we want to make in this book is that *stigma should not be used in any way, for any reason, to promote public health.* Doctors shouldn't be quietly shaming obese patients to motivate them to exercise more. Development workers shouldn't be shaming people into building toilets, either. That gets in the way of what they are there to do in the first place—help communities thrive.

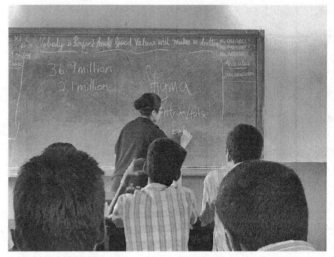

Figure C.1. Arizona State University global health students in Chennai, India, 2017, assisting with anti-HIV/AIDS stigma programs. Photo by A. Brewis

Shame in all its forms needs to be removed from the public health tool kit, because it too easily misfires.

Some may argue that stigma evolved to keep people healthy when avoidance was the only way to prevent disease, so it remains legitimate to deploy it in public health efforts, like triggering Community-Led Total Sanitation or dissuading consumption of sugar-sweetened beverages. Regardless, it doesn't matter. The conditions of modern-day society and healthcare are nothing like the social conditions in which humans evolved. Solutions that worked back then are quite obviously inadequate and inappropriate today. In small-scale societies, using stigma to socially isolate a few "undesirables" may have resulted in personal tragedies—lives lost and wasted—but they did not have the capacity to create large-scale social inequalities and suffering. In our own complexly structured societies, stigmatization deepens and entrenches massive, systemic injustices, harming our health, our economy, and the quality of all our lives.

We have other health promoting options anyway—ones that avoid the problem of creating stigma altogether. Public health strategies, ranging from hospital isolation units to sick days at work, to do the work of distancing us from disease more effectively than stigma ever could. Public health messaging can motivate behavior by using social desirability and pro-social incentives. It is likely to be just as effective, for instance, to design health messaging that suggests people make an effort not to be "forgetful" about using a condom so they don't hurt others, rather than suggesting non-condom use means they are being stupid, dangerous, or malicious.[1] Patients respond far better to empathetic caregivers than to judgment and disapproval. Underfunded and overworked healthcare providers around the world already have enough trouble connecting with patients—stigmatizing messages just further weaken the sadly tenuous bond between patients and caregivers.

It is morally right and tactically important to destigmatize global health practice, but that does not mean it will be easy. One of the greatest challenges is that every decision made in medicine and global health has the potential to create *more* stigma harm. One reason for this is that the social human brain is designed to judge and does so quickly and easily. Those who stigmatize, especially when they have power like that provided by the medical establishment, may not be immediately aware of what they are doing. Or if they are, they don't feel any discomfort or guilt because the words or action that follow just feel normal, right, and natural. Moreover, stigmas tend to intersect and cluster. Those who hold socially devalued roles with much less power (such as women, racial and ethnic minorities, immigrants, people living in poverty) are often more likely to develop stigmatized health conditions *and* more likely to be blamed for them. This greatly complicates professionals' capacity to see and react to stigma in ways that help. Even the most well-meaning professionals can make assumptions—culturally common beliefs but medically wrong inferences—about people's motivations, behaviors, and circumstances.

The unquestioned nature of stigma, embedded in our norms as what feels "normal and right," is what makes it so insidious. Wrong assumptions can lead well-meaning professionals to design treatments and interventions that reinforce intersecting stigmas, rather than advance the destigmatization work that medicine and global health so desperately need. So how can global health professionals, who are mostly not stigma researchers and may not have time or opportunity for an eight-week training course, identify and counteract hidden and intersecting stigmas in health programs? We have developed a short checklist to help evaluate the likelihood of stigma in any intervention, proposed policy, or medical consultation (table C.1).

If you checked any of the items, you are working with a social group or global health problem that is at high risk of highly damaging forms of stigma. You should think very carefully about the way the global health program, public health intervention, or medical consultation is designed to ensure that it does not inadvertently shame or blame people whose health is at risk, and that best practices for building provider-patient communication and rapport are followed. This means showing respect for patients (no matter who they are or what they can afford to pay), making an effort to build trust, communicating with people in ways they value and understand, and engaging caregivers and communities in patient care and health outreach.

If you checked two or more boxes, we recommend that your global health program, public health intervention, or medical consultation should have an *explicit destigmatization approach*. Given the presence of two or more existing stigmas, our work indicates that—even if the program promotes no stigmatizing messages—it is extremely likely that (1) health workers will inadvertently convey stigmatizing messages in the delivery of neutral health or medical content or (2) patients or beneficiaries will implicitly perceive stigmatizing messages, as these are embedded in their typical day-to-day interactions.

Addressing stigma within existing global health programming should always be done at the local level, in ways that speak to the specific concerns, priorities and understandings of the patients or community.[2] The ILEP Guidelines to Reduce Stigma (of leprosy) are some of the most cogent in this regard.[3] They lay out steps for assessing leprosy stigma, using locally relevant quantitative and qualitative methods to identify what stigma exists on the ground and suggest different procedures for testing public versus self-stigma. We recom-

TABLE C.1.
Stigma checklist for interventions, policies, or consultations

Social indicators	Examples
Is the patient or target population . . .	
primarily composed of people in vulnerable gender or age groups?	Women, girls, boys, elderly
primarily composed of people identifying as LGBTQ+ or sexual minorities?	Lesbian, gay, transgender, non-binary
a marginalized racial, ethnic, or religious group?	Black and indigenous people in the United States, Muslims in Europe
part of a group characterized by low, highly unstable, and/or non-legal income?	Itinerant/undocumented farm workers, garbage pickers, recipients of public assistance, sex workers
part of a group characterized by lack of adequate access to basic amenities/resources?	People living in very low-income neighborhoods, food- or water-insecure communities
one that speaks a different language from the rest of the society, has high rates of illiteracy, or does not understand the formal language of government?	Asylum seekers in Australia, Quechua speakers in South America, non-French speakers in Haiti

Health indicators	Examples
Does the health risk or medical condition . . .	
have a risk profile that is often called "cultural"?	Domestic violence, alcohol abuse
have a risk profile related to poor living conditions?	Malnutrition, cholera
have a behavioral component, through which those at risk are commonly blamed for their own illness?	Obesity, lung cancer, HIV
have an association with patients considered socially undesirable or problematic?	Drug addiction, mental illness
qualify as a complex, poorly understood condition that is difficult to diagnose and treat?	Fibromyalgia, chronic fatigue syndrome, autism/ASD, infertility

TABLE C.2.
Some basic destigmatization strategies

Relabel	Give the condition a new name
Reframe	Remove blame, often emphasizing biological causes
Reeducate	Expose popular misconceptions and reduce fear
Connect	Meet with real patients, show them as valuable people with full lives
Advocate	Social activism, public disclosure, community building
Build Self-Esteem	Help stigma sufferers reject self-stigma

mend these guidelines as a solid starting point for any teams wanting to design better approaches that take these factors into account. The general approach is suitable for tackling many types of stigma, not just leprosy.

The more tools in the tool kit, the better. To recap, these are the tactics that can be deployed in anti-stigma efforts, each discussed in some depth in this book (table C.2). Although these are the best available anti-stigma approaches developed over many years to combat stigma, it's important to note, too, that none of them have really solid evidence—collected over time or across cultures—to suggest that they will actually work in all the many complex, dynamic contexts of global health. In fact, we have presented cases in the book where each of these approaches has failed in some destructive way, regardless of the best intentions. It is safe to say that even partly successful destigmatization effort will likely need to be working through multiple means and at multiple levels: family, community, and institutional.[4]

In some situations, such as an unfolding infectious epidemic of Ebola or H1N1 influenza, there is little time to study and test all options. Immediate action is required. The strategies to destigmatize need to be developed and applied quickly and need constant reassessment and adjustment. In such cases, we highly recommend calling in anthropologists who can move quickly to extract the key cultural information and transform it into action.

This approach is increasingly used in real-world global health crises—and it's a proven success. Our medical anthropologist colleague, Sharon Abramowitz, has done long-term fieldwork in Liberia in Western Africa, where the recent Ebola outbreak was concentrated.

In 2014, Abramowitz was passionately working to coordinate the American Anthropological Association / Emergency Ebola Anthropology Initiative (figure C.2). In the main city of Monrovia, during the accelerating outbreak, she demonstrated that properly developed and delivered public health messages could rapidly spread in ways that would quickly reduce fear and forestall further infection.[5]

Despite such successes, there isn't yet as much uptake as we need in global health organizations. In 2014, at the height of the Ebola crisis, Abramowitz documented the details of a phone call she made to the New York City office of Médecins Sans Frontières (Doctors Without Borders):[6]

> *Abramowitz:* Hi. I'm a medical anthropologist with fourteen years of experience studying healthcare, health systems, and humanitarian aid in Guinea, Liberia, and Côte d'Ivoire. I heard your director put out a call for help on Ebola on NPR today, and I really think I can help you.
>
> *Médecins Sans Frontières:* I'm sorry, but we don't work with medical anthropologists in general, except for under very rare circumstances.

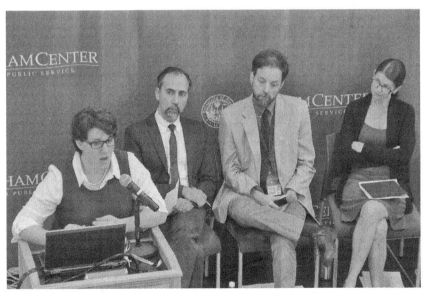

Figure C.2. Medical anthropologist Sharon Abramowitz advocating for a more culturally appropriate response to the Ebola outbreak in Liberia, 2014. Courtesy of S. Abramowitz

If you really want to help out Doctors Without Borders, you are going to have to go to our website to register as a volunteer. The process takes nine to twelve months, and even if we decide that we need your skills, we still won't guarantee that you will go to the country where you have done research. But please understand that it's extremely rare that we ever have a need for a medical anthropologist.

How Do We Make Stigma More Visible?

To tackle the pernicious effects of stigma on human health, we also need to render its scale and impacts fully apparent. By making stigma more visible, we mean two things. First, most global health practitioners know that stigma is a bad thing, but view it mostly as a side issue—just one of a myriad of impediments to preventing and treating specific conditions like HIV/AIDS or epilepsy. Second, there is little understanding of stigma's pervasive power, operating as a silent but deadly force creating widespread illness. This is because we aren't orienting our global health efforts in the right ways to reveal this. We aren't even identifying and tracking stigma as part of normal global health efforts.

In the early 2000s, Mitchell Weiss and his colleagues laid an important agenda for how to advance these goals through the application of solid social science and epidemiological research.[7] Yet, as our anthropologist colleagues Emily Mendenhall, Kristin Yarris, and Brandon Kohrt recently pointed out in an essay, too few scholars today use the full tool kit. By a tool kit, we mean the full range of research methods that can help us understand stigma and its impacts.[8] So, we suggest that revisiting, updating, and expanding Weiss's practical suggestions is a great place to start to make stigma more visible.

Step 1: Increase Practitioner Awareness

To begin, we need to make global health practitioners sufficiently aware of ways stigma can undermine their efforts, and then we can provide the tools to be able to better foresee and forestall it. This book is an effort in that direction. In the field of epidemiology, the role of stigma as a crucial driver of population health must be clearly highlighted. A number of important efforts in this regard have begun. But in our conversations with people trained in traditional medical models (such as the behavior-change model in public health), many seem to find it difficult to imagine that stigma is much more than a peripheral aspect of human illness. Rendering stigma and its damage visible requires health professionals to be able to more easily and readily identify it in their everyday working lives.

This perspective is a product of a medical training system that focuses on proximate rather than ultimate causes of illness. Shifting health training is the right place to begin. More medical schools are considering some form of "structural competency" training within their curriculum. The approach shifts the clinician's view to recognizing how health disparities are produced through social and institutional disadvantages. It steps well away from the notion that illness is produced by individuals' (often poor) own decisions, emphasizing instead how people's decision-making is profoundly constrained by their economic, political, and social environment.

Universities and medical residencies can play an important role in helping health professionals recognize the biases and limitations of their medical training and personal experiences.[9] Stigma is an outstanding example of how these biases work. We have been applying case studies at the intersection of stigma and poverty at the core of our global health undergraduate curriculum at Arizona State University for some years,[10] and we see it is creating health professionals with the capacity to see stigma for what it is. The goal is to help a new generation of structurally sensitive health professionals navigate the often unfamiliar, complex, and interconnected constraints and vulnerabilities their stigmatized patients face.

Joseph (Joe) Canarie is a former student of ours who exemplifies how such forms of training can benefit both doctors and their patients. When Joe was an undergraduate in ASU's Global Health program, he designed a unique research project to explore transgender people's experiences of homelessness. Working closely with our team, he learned new techniques for doing ethical ethnographic research with vulnerable LGBTQ+ populations. After graduating from ASU, Joe continued on to medical school at Dartmouth University. Today, he is a resident physician in pediatric and internal medicine at Yale New Haven Hospital. He also serves as an advisor on LGBTQ+ Affairs, contributing his expertise on transgender children's medical needs to medical student training.

Another goal of our program, and others like it, is to enculturate the idea that destigmatization is a form of social justice activism that must underlie all highly effective healthcare. In our own classes, we have started testing which forms of instruction around stigma and discrimination have the most impact on global health students' awareness of structural barriers, such as caused by racial, ethnic, gender, and age discrimination.[11] One important proposed aspect of this emerging area of "structural competency" training to promote sufficient humility to appreciate the crucial systemic change mostly happens slowly, requiring long-term effort and broad collaborations with affected communities.[12] Our hope is that this will shape how this new generation of health professionals who are particularly well-equipped to advance health as a human right throughout their careers.

For mental health stigma, psychiatrists are arguably the set of health professionals who can do the most to help. Our colleague Brandon Kohrt, who is a psychiatrist-anthropologist and global health expert, found in his fieldwork in Nepal that local "stigma systems"—how people recognize and react to what is normal or not in a specific cultural context—may overlap from place to place in useful ways.[13] This thinking laid the groundwork for his work in designing the George Washington University's innovative, eight-week training program for resident psychiatrists. In this program, stigma is understood as "an affliction of normal people and normal brains." It should always be expected and planned for.[14] Thus, core modules include how to anticipate and manage mental health stigma in the clinic and family settings, helping patients identify and cope with internalized stigma, and working around the stigma of medical colleagues, families, communities and patients themselves. Here, Kohrt and his colleagues are making the key point that destigmatization is not just a moral imperative; it's a basic requirement for creating high-quality psychiatric healthcare.

Step 2: Track Stigma

We need to be doing a better job of tracking levels of stigma as they vary from place to place and change through time. The good news is that we can use epidemiological and social science forms of evidence gathering to achieve this goal. Doing so will help us address questions such as: Who is most at risk, both in terms of public stigma exposure and the internalization of stigma (as the most damaging form of self-stigma)? And, why? Which health interventions worsen stigma, either intentionally or unintentionally? What forms of stigma interventions are most effective?

The successes and failures of destigmatization efforts themselves need to be tracked, too. Much effort has been put into fighting against single stigmas as part of a broader strategy for solving specific disease problems, like HIV/AIDS and mental illness. However, not enough has been done to track the long-term impacts of these efforts.[15] In other words, we don't yet know what works to quell stigma over the long term in the real world, even in the best studied cases (like HIV or leprosy). And, as we explored in part III, stigmas tend to cluster together and the compounding effects of each can be very hard to disentangle. We need to develop and use validated instruments that capture the felt impacts of general and compounded effects of stigmas. Tracking one stigma at a time will always be insufficient.

A good example of how to begin comes from obesity research. We have clues that weight-loss interventions are promoting new stigmas— ones that actually make it harder to lose weight. Although fat activists had been sounding the alarm, few scholars were making efforts to track how much stigma people feel before, during, and after interventions.

To address this in our research with weight-loss surgery patients at the Mayo Clinic, we measured levels of stigma on standard psychometric scales. Ostensibly, stigma should drop off with the pounds. However, the results show that weight stigma persists even as people lose weight after bariatric surgeries. Moreover, that stigma makes it harder for patients to follow the complex postsurgical dietary rules, such as only eating small amounts and having protein at the start of every meal.[16] We suspect higher levels of residual felt stigma play a role in explaining which patients are most likely to regain weight years later. Better tracking, in this way, will help us gather evidence for what works, what doesn't, and why.

Tracking stigma meaningfully isn't just about quantifying it—figuring how much stigma there is and how many people are affected. We must also understand the quality of stigma experiences—what it is, what it is doing to people, and how this differs based on where someone sits in the social hierarchy.[17] Such work demands a more explicitly ethnographic approach to our anti-stigma efforts. For example, destigmatization efforts must be evaluated not just by how much stigma people are exposed to. They must also assess where those most affected by stigma are socially located, and the level of harm and dysfunction people experience in their daily lives as a result.

Stigma tracking must be grounded in local knowledge and experiences. This means examining what matters most[18] for people locally, given that the forms stigma takes can change from place to place. We need to ask: On what basis do people think they are being judged by others? When and how does this bother them? How does this manifest in specific social hierarchies? When does stigma translate into distress or otherwise harm people? Where and how do they find ways to cope and overcome?

Ethnographies are often the best way to answer questions about how people construct and live in worlds of meaning. Ethnographies are especially powerful ways to present the profound emotional misery of living with stigmatized labels. Two examples we often recommend to our students are Loïc Wacquant's work on urban marginality and Joan Ablon's work on physical disability.

French sociologist Loïc Wacquant's work on "urban outcasts"[19] began when he was listening to French and American officials talk with similar disgust about the people living in their public housing projects. Drawing on Erving Goffman's work about how stigma is created, Wacquant provides a compelling account of what he metaphorically calls the "leprous badlands." The French stigmatized neighborhoods, and the stigmatized people they contained, were viewed as a product of the overextension of the welfare state. The US neighborhoods were created by racialized segregation, criminalization, and denial of welfare to Black people. But the overall story has major similarities in both cases. Political and social systems, constructed and propelled by stigma, act to marginalize and victimize the people living in them.

Joan Ablon was an anthropologist trained in the 1950s–1960s who worked in many of the same contexts we have—in rural Mexico, with Samoans, and in the southwestern United States. With this global perspective, she was one of the first social scientists to recognize and articulate the recurring links between being labeled with illness or a disability, being on the outskirts of society, and being stigmatized.[20] Later in her career, she wrote a compelling ethnography of people of very short stature in the United States.[21] She explains through this case how stigmas attached to the most deeply held moral values become those that damage the most. In the United States, where height is a core value associated with leadership, attractiveness, and capability, the genetic condition of dwarfism pushes you down and out of society, triggering both practical and emotional difficulties. Her work explains in vivid detail how the world just isn't built to fit, or always willing to include, the least tall members of society.

At the same time, detailed ethnographic narratives help us understand in powerful ways the *costs* that accrue to groups of people who become targets of stigma. And more—and here we come back to our deeper sense of optimism—ethnographies have also provided compelling portraits of how stigmatized individuals and groups have found hope and improved their lives. Ablon explains how the efforts of the organization Little People of America has created spaces for resisting stigma. A careful read of such ethnographies can provide important information as we seek to create destigmatization strategies that have a better chance of success. They are also one of the best ways to build empathy, which is a powerful way to break down stereotypes and can open up new, needed conversations to challenge stigma.

Step 3: Connect Evidence to Policy

To make awareness matter, we need to better connect academic and applied findings on stigma to policy. Wacquant centered this in his scholarly writing, pointedly examining how urban housing was being mishandled by a stigmatizing government.[22] But we need to find ways to move these ideas more directly to effective action.

We need better and more easily available scientific proof of how and why some groups are more affected than others. This will make it easier for people in stigmatized situations to argue for policies and practices that reduce burdens on the more vulnerable members of society.[23] Many people working in global health are well-situated to help with this challenge, including journalists, activists, healthcare workers, development workers, advocacy groups, and, of course, our elected officials.

Anthropologist-physician Paul Farmer is an inspiring example of this principle in action: He has spent decades using ethnographic stories to inform the medical establishment about the relationship between stigma, infectious disease, and poverty in Haiti. His work pushes for changes in the way health efforts are implemented on the ground.[24] But, frustrated by the lack of adequate institutional action, he worked with four colleagues to start Partners In Health, a medical charity in Haiti, in 1987. Now working with community organizations in ten countries, Partners In Health provides medical care in ways that destigmatize and provide a preferential option for the poor.

With stigma all around us, it is impossible to combat every form of stigma at all times. We need the right tools to address those stigmas that are most damaging. We must differentiate what merely causes transitory discomfort or slight embarrassment from that which is relentlessly, mortifyingly, emotionally devastating. For example, the policy that tells people they cannot smoke in public places is not nearly as damaging as the policies that deny the poorest among us (who are more likely to smoke) from having adequate healthcare coverage.

After decades of field research, we believe the most damage is done by stigmas that particularly target the socially disadvantaged and marginalized. Good examples of this are the cases of leprosy and cholera, which we discussed in chapter 2. These stigmas destroy lives and rip apart the fabric of societies. This is where we need to start our most serious and focused work. If we do this well, we will also learn how to combat the smaller, less destructive stigmas that make everyone's lives more difficult and less healthy as well.

I Don't Work in Global Health. What Can I Do?

Changing how we deliver healthcare is only part of the solution. The rest has to come from all of us, in our everyday lives. But what can we do to help, if we don't work in public health, development, or public policy?

Because stigma is so ubiquitous in our lives, each of us has the chance to act against and challenge it every single day. One place to start is to support legislation that provides basic protection and dignity to everyone. In the United States, providing high-quality universal healthcare would go a long way in addressing stigma-related denial of care. In addition, antidiscrimination legislation, too, is much needed. Weight discrimination, as we discussed in part III, remains perfectly legal even as other forms of discrimination are outlawed.

Even without legislation, the harm of stigma can be mitigated by creating socially valued roles where people with stigmatized identities can thrive. The case of mental health covered in part II showed—as with married women with schizophrenia in Palau, Micronesia, and depressed migrant men from Nepal—the availability of socially valued roles can make or break people's lives. Many of these roles will be related to work opportunities, simply because productive roles are universally valued. In this way, nonprofit efforts to train those on the autism spectrum to succeed in the new software development professions are absolutely on point. Similarly, efforts to provide decent paid work for people with other types of mental or physical challenges are a powerful way to contribute.

Not all socially valued roles need be in the realm of paid labor. Becoming woven into the fabric of their society greatly matters for people to enjoy a sense of belonging and dignity. Being able to marry and raise children allows people to occupy the valued social roles of cherished spouses and loving parents. Serving one's community, through work in a voluntary or religious organization, allows people to build social networks of mutual support. Housing that is nonsegregated, affordable, and accessible allows people to take on the social role of good neighbors. And being an activist—working to fight stigma and change society—is an incredibly important, valuable, and often personally rewarding social role.

For those who are themselves the targets of stigma, finding others who have similar experiences can be another powerful step to combatting it. Erving Goffman talked about the value of what he called "sympathetic others"—people who know or otherwise understand and relate to our pain because they share it. By locating support groups, reaching out to others, and bravely sharing our stories, there is the potential for awareness, action, and change. For those living with stigma, there is already a large set of materials around how to reach out for help and support. The internet now is brimming with supportive materials, ideas, and groups to connect with. Many of these focus around a single health condition like tuberculosis, obesity, mental illness, or HIV.

One of the challenges with this approach is that sometimes connecting in powerful ways with other sympathetic stigma-sharers causes the stigma to define us even more. Consider our recent research on weight-loss bloggers, which showed that blogging empowered and helped them connect to others who could support them but also exposed them to vicious internet trolls.[25] Moreover, many people at the bottom of the social hierarchy who struggle most with stigma are least

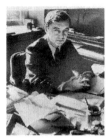

Figure C.3. Erving Goffman at his desk. Source unknown.

able to connect with these types of support networks. They don't have the time or resources. Solving stigma is never a simple, one-step solution. Like stigma itself, it's more of a process, and one that demands amazing bravery and resolve.

So, the support of friends and family matters greatly. By supporting people and encouraging them to engage with so-called communities of suffering, everyone can make a real and crucial difference. Goffman highlighted the importance of stigma solutions that connect those living with stigma to what he called "wise others." These are people who don't carry the stigma but who empathize and can provide support as a fellow traveler for those that do. This can be complicated, since some of the most painful stigma interactions arise from the judgments of those closest to us, such as family, colleagues, and classmates. But these are the people who can also most help.

We are not saying any of this is easy. When we resist expressing stigma we are fighting some of our core, evolved human tendencies to judge others. Even Erving Goffman himself (figure C.3), no less than the preeminent stigma scholar of all time, had trouble applying his theoretical positions to those he interacted with most in his daily life. After his death, many of his former colleagues and students were interviewed at length to better document his life and work. One described his take-no-prisoners approach:

> There was a badly crippled woman in the class yet he persisted in talking about "gimps." There was also a student with a severe stuttering problem. This did not prevent her from asking ques-

tions. Acting as if she was not present, Goffman offered material
which was sometimes humorous about how stutterers managed
(e.g., by taking jobs as night watchmen). He reduced another female
student to tears during an office hour meeting. He was critical of her
ideas and told her he did not think women should be in graduate
school. At the end of the last class session a black student said, "This is
all very interesting Professor Goffman, but what's the use of it for
changing the conditions you describe?" He stood up, slammed shut the
book he had open on the desk and said "I'm not in that business" and
stormed out of the room. During an open meeting in the midst of one
Berkeley crisis or another [in the early 1960s], someone said "Professor
Goffman, where do you stand?" He responded, "When they start
shooting students from the steps of Sproul Hall I guess I'll get involved,
but not until then." I recall being stunned.[26]

A major takeaway from this book, then, is that stigma is always
going to be fundamental to the human condition. We need to approach stigma reduction with profound humility, and a deep understanding that our first responsibility must be to minimize the harm
that we ourselves do. Stigma is something we all are making either
worse or better through every interaction.

We are cultural beings who take on and reflect the values of the
societies to which we belong. Thus, many stigmas slip in unnoticed or
are enacted without any cost or guilt to those who express them. We
are all a little Goffman-like at some level—incredibly good at judging
everyone we come across, finding them lacking, and finding defensi-
bility in our reaction. If we are not actively considering our choices, it
is easy to hire "that nice boy" because we know just by looking at him
that he will work harder. Or it is easy to laugh when the fat kid gets
teased. Or think it is okay to want to keep someone with HIV out of
our dorm or neighborhood, because they may be dangerous or otherwise morally dubious.

In these everyday decisions and actions, together we create and reinforce stigma. To undo this stigma, we need to accept those defined
as different and less valuable. These actions are mostly small and

simple in the moment. We can resist telling loved ones with mental illness to "man up" or "get over it." We can modify how we react to strangers unlike us at the mall or the airport, and try to avoid obvious signs of judgment like staring or making snide comments or laughing. We can muster our courage, too, and tell those who shame others that it is unacceptable. Noticing stigma and working to address it in each of our daily lives builds better communities for all of us. It can have positive impacts on everyone around us, ourselves included.

Just *noticing* our own stigmatizing thoughts and behaviors is the first, and sometimes trickiest, crucial step. Often, we only notice our own stigmas when prevailing social attitudes change and like-minded friends no longer surround us. We might be criticized for our out-of-touch views of same-sex marriage. Or we may find ourselves in a lawsuit when our practiced behaviors suddenly illegally exclude people with disabilities. Goffman would have been horrified, we hope, to read his colleagues' accounts of how his interpersonal style wrought such damage on others. We can try to do a bit better.

Knowing that social norms can change—and becoming a part of the vanguard making that change happen—is the next step. We need to get better at catching our own stigma, while it is still socially acceptable, and work harder toward destigmatization. Cultural norms can change slowly, one interaction at a time. That means that every effort we make to destigmatize our thoughts, speech, and actions really can count. We can be more aware of the ways we communicate our negative judgments to others and really try to temper them. If nothing else, this will make our own small social networks happier and healthier.

If we learn a final lesson from Erving Goffman—that very complicated hero and antihero of stigma—it should be this: Knowledge about stigma isn't enough. We need empathy and action, too. Harnessed, it can create anti-stigma power—a force with the capacity to help heal us all.

Stigma
A Brief Primer

What Is Stigma?

Stigma is best viewed as a *process* rather than a thing.[1] Through the process of being stigmatized, people become socially stained and discredited because they hold a characteristic that is classified as unacceptable or undesirable.[2] They lose social standing and become viewed as "less than." They are then moved out, down, or away from society. In this sense, stigma is about the *consequences* of a failure to meet prevailing social norms. Human dignity is something we all value and seek. Stigma is the opposite—it is a force that strips away our social status and self-worth. This is because at the heart of most stigmatizing processes is the belief that people are to be *blamed* and *shamed* (their fault) or *pitied* (not their fault) for having the characteristic.

The effect of stigma is strongest when *moral* meanings are attached to that failure. For example, in the United States, people with disabilities are stigmatized when they cannot meet cultural norms of autonomy and independence. People with leprous skin lesions were defined in European history as not just diseased but also unclean and immoral, and they were ostracized as a result. Similarly, people living with obesity are increasingly stigmatized by associations of body fat with laziness, lack of self-control, and other devalued moral characteristics. Thus, even though obese bodies are increasingly common (now one-third of adults in many countries), the "fat" body is still defined as an abnormal one. This supports teasing, bullying, and other forms of rejection and discrimination as socially acceptable.

Forms of Stigma

Among academics, stigma is divided into a number of subtypes. *Public stigma* refers to the widespread, approved ways that stigmatizing ideas and actions are evident in our everyday lives. Widespread public stigma reflects broad social agreement that the stereotype is true, that the negative judgment is correct, and that discriminatory action seems warranted.

Public stigma can be communicated in a myriad of ways: the punchline in a sitcom, schoolyard bullying, the "helpful" nagging of a family member, a doctor's questions, the trouble you have getting a job or an apartment, the averted gaze of strangers when you are out in public, or the image on a public health poster.[3] When stigma turns into action in these ways, it is sometimes termed *enacted stigma*.[4]

Sometimes the signs we direct outward to others are communicating a judgment or prejudice that we are fully or vaguely aware of (our *explicit stigma*). Other times they happen outside of our self-awareness because we are just doing what feels normal, natural, and expected (our *implicit stigma*).[5] This becomes *felt stigma* when the people who are the targets of explicit or implicit stigma become *aware* of prejudicial attitudes and notice the stigma enacted toward them. It need not be acts directly experienced, either. Hearing stories of mistreatment by other people who are similar to us, such as other people with the same disease, makes us feel stigma too.

Structural stigma refers to stigma that is created and reinforced by institutions such as governments, medical practice, schools, businesses, or community associations. For example, people with high body weights find the physical environments of public spaces, such as airline seats, deliberately exclude them. Similarly, research funding or insurance coverage for drug addiction is seen as less important than for other diseases (like breast cancer or childhood leukemia) where people are considered blameless for their affliction.

Self-stigma is the most personally damaging form of stigma, because it has profound emotional power. It is the internalization of public stigma in ways that push us to question and devalue our core identities. Self-stigma happens when people are aware they are being stigmatized, they agree the negative judgment has merit, and they apply it to themselves. For example, people struggling with obesity may notice public stigma toward people with obesity and agree that fat people are lazy and ugly. They would then conclude, "I am fat; therefore, I too am lazy and ugly." You can feel stigma without then self-stigmatizing ("I may be fat, but I disagree that means I am lazy or ugly.") or you can self-stigmatize without feeling stigma ("I am fat and I agree that fat people are lazy—but I don't believe that others are judging me for it.").

Courtesy stigma is when others connected to the stigmatized are also themselves socially discredited by association. Healthcare workers in aged-care facilities are themselves stained by managing the "disgusting" incontinence of residents,[6] and those working with people with disabilities are viewed as having no quality of life or job satisfaction. Courtesy stigma can extend to families too, such as parents with HIV-positive children who are judged as having raised someone who was sexually indiscriminate or a drug user.

How Does Stigma Work?

To explain in more detail how stigma is created and perpetuated, here we identify eight core theoretical understandings that explain current thinking and that are reflected in the presentation of cases throughout the book.

1. Stigma is embedded in our cultural norms and values.

Stigma is one possible result of failing to meet prevailing public *cultural norms*. By norms, we mean what people generally and collectively agree is normal, acceptable, or desirable. The hygiene norms discussed in chapters 1 and 2 are a good example of this. In places such as the United States, United Kingdom, and Canada, handwashing after using the bathroom is a *norm*—everyone is *expected* to do it. Norms need not exactly match what people actually do. Many people don't always wash their hands, even if they know it is the *right* thing to do.

These types of judgmental norms that define stigma become attached to any number of characteristics. They may be identifiable by body characteristics: visible tooth decay, being too hairy or too bald, being too short, or in a wheelchair. They can be applied to behaviors that may not be directly observed: drinking alcohol, sexual indiscrimination, or bulimic vomiting. They attach easily to a diagnosis with an undesirable or little understood condition: epilepsy, HIV, or prostate cancer. The stigmatized trait need not even actually exist. It must only be *perceived* to exist.

Stigmas tend to be strongest where people are seen as *morally* responsible for their condition; overweight people may be seen as lazy or unmotivated or people who test HIV positive may be seen as sexually promiscuous or using illegal drugs. Where disease is seen as outside of one's own control, a twist of fate, or just bad luck, stigma tends to be softer and easier to manage. Yet even though some conditions carry less moral blame—like blindness or Alzheimer's or epilepsy—they can draw pity. The assumption that pitiful people have no quality of life can add to the felt stigma because it also allows and encourages social distancing and exclusion.

This close association between stigma and blaming people for their condition also explains why discriminatory treatment by others (such as teasing or bullying), especially when enacted within institutions (like quarantine laws for leprosy), are seen within mainstream society to be both appropriate and justified. Queen Elizabeth I is said to have bathed about once a month—about as often as Doña Maria from Bolivia, who we introduced in chapter 3. But smelling bad was not seen as a moral transgression in Elizabethan England. It was instead viewed as a practical reality that transcended classes, and thus, it wasn't as socially damaging.

Stigmas always make local sense. They map onto, remind, and reinforce our *core* social values.[7] For example, as we discussed in chapter 9, the symptoms associated with severe depression—like social withdrawal and thoughts of suicide—are a great concern in all societies. But the basic *reasons* for why they are so socially threatening, and hence who they most stigmatize, differ. In China, where preserving family lineage was historically a core concern, depression in unmarried adults might be concerning if it is seen to undermine the ability of the family to engage in the types of social relationships (like marriage) that are needed to meet this social goal. In contrast, in Latin America, depression in married men might be worrisome if it suggests someone is unable to fulfil the patriarchal role of provider and protector of the family.

The way stigma applies may be different by gender, ethnicity, income, or age based on social roles. A man carrying herpes or human papilloma virus might be judged as a "player," whereas a woman with the same disease is more likely to be judged as sexually indiscriminate and "damaged goods." An elderly person with extra body weight is more acceptable than a younger one, because some weight gain is seen as a "normal" part of aging.

Stigmas are also dynamic. They change through time. Diseases, it seems, are most likely to be stigmatized when they have no known cause nor cure.[8] Advances in medical knowledge can, thus, be very influential. Leprosy stigma decreased markedly when the bacteria causing the disease was identified and better therapies were developed. In prior generations, breast cancer was surrounded by shame and secrecy, but, with new treatments and a better prognosis, it has shifted from being seen as a death sentence to a heroic fight for life.

2. Stigma is created and reinforced both institutionally and interpersonally.

Illnesses don't stigmatize people; people and the institutions they create do.[9] Stigmas, and the norms that permit them, are created and reinforced every day. People aren't stigmatized *because* of having HIV or leprosy or chlamydia; they are stigmatized by the thoughts, speech, and actions of people around them. Stigma is communicated in the words we choose ("fat," "retarded," "gimp"); in mocking, teasing, and physical bullying; and by cruel postings on social media. It is created when we avoid a gaze, look away, or cross the street. It is reinforced when we take longer to serve someone in a shop or to treat them in an emergency room. It is embedded in the choices made when a landlord rents an apartment, a boss offers a promotion, a teacher calls on someone in class, or peers decide where to sit during lunchtime. Because stigmatizing thoughts, speech, and actions align so closely with barely questioned core cultural values, people colluding in this everyday production of stigma often consider their behavior fully justified. They also may not be fully aware of the messages they are sending because it just feels like business as usual.

Institutions like media, law, religion, industry, and government communicate and reinforce stigma, too. Churches decide who "deserves" charity. Our governments determine who should be quarantined for public safety, denied treatment to spare the public purse, or allowed access based on their disabilities. "Fashionable" stores don't offer clothing in larger sizes, and "standard" seat belts and seats on airplanes fail to fit many comfortably, reminding people that it is unacceptable to be large. Employers decide comfortable breastfeeding facilities aren't important, forcing women to pump their breastmilk in toilet stalls or to give up breastfeeding—or working—altogether. Television presents images in ways that reinforce the superiority of such traits as youth, slimness, and elevated mood over being older, fatter, or depressed. News stories reinforce the idea that low-income, minority, and immigrant neighborhoods are dangerous and less deserving, shaping fewer government investments in the provision of green space, hospitals, pollution mitigation, and policing. This then adds to the likelihood that people in such neighborhoods will get or stay hurt or sick.

3. Diseases are particular magnet for stigma.

Global health is one of the ripest areas for studying stigma processes. This is because disease is a particularly strong magnet for them. Illness is one of the shared conditions that all humans worry about, and the most damaging stigmas reflect and feed on what people care about. Those permutations of "what matters most" are culturally defined.

Mental illness is more likely to be stigmatized, as we discussed in chapter 8, when it interferes with culturally defined "productive" social roles, such as holding down a nine-to-five job or getting married. Moreover, disease follows and reinforces poverty, and a whole host of other intersecting vulnerabilities as we discussed in chapter 9. Stigma can become an easy tool for signaling fear or distrust, as we explained in chapter 3, and so a common lever for pushing people further down and out in society.

Diseases that are considered contagious and deadly evoke the most fear. Contagious diseases are more likely to evoke pernicious stigmas, such as the cholera epidemics discussed in chapter 3. Diseases with less hope of permanent recovery also tend to be a focus of persistent stigma, such as the case of schizophrenia detailed in chapters 7 and 8. The introduction of modern pharmaceutical treatments for tuberculosis, leprosy, and HIV/AIDS have all been helpful in reducing fears about the disease and accordingly its stigma. Those diseases where moral failings are generally believed the central causes of disease (such as laziness and lack of self-control in obesity, or sinful indulgence in addiction or sexually transmitted diseases) tend to be more stigmatizing than those where moral fault is considered absent, a point clearly made in chapter 5.

Stigma and medicalization, the shift to conditions being defined by and treated via medical knowledge and practice, have a complex dynamic. Labeling conditions as disease and recognizing or preferring medical treatments can both variously increase and decrease risk of stigma for the affected person, as explored in chapter 7 on mental illness. The stigma of addiction has reduced with growing recognition of it as a somewhat treatable medical disease, in part because this shifts away the notion of personal blame in the etiology of the related alcohol abuse or drug use. In our own research, we have seen how parents of "badly behaved" schoolchildren often find a diagnosis of ADHD is useful not only to their children's school performance and provision of better services, but also their own sense of their worth as parents as blame shifts from them to "genetics."[10] Yet, a child's diagnosis can also bring new felt courtesy stigma to the parent also, such as believing others judge the use of psychoactive drugs as a crutch for their poor parenting.[11]

Similarly, bariatric patients in our studies with Mayo Clinic patients have revealed how important demonstrating to everyone around them that they are medically compliant (such as exercising regularly) is crucial to controlling the stigmatization they experience from others around them.[12]

However, sometimes defining a medical condition or getting a diagnosis can itself create or reinforce stigma. For example, as we showed in chapter 6, increasing efforts to address obesity as a medical condition seem to be only exaggerating the stigma and resulting suffering, in part because the medical approach emphasizes weight as an index of personal failure. Diagnosis with a severe mental illness can trigger new stigma, exactly because it now has a name, as we explained in chapter 4. And, to add to the complex relationship between stigma and disease, sometimes playing into and embracing stigmas can in itself *reduce* the social or physical suffering of disease and help with treatment. Shared stigma suffering can bring people together in ways that connect them, so the very experience of the stigma in turn becomes part of their healing.[13]

4. Coping with and resisting stigma is hard work.

People do not just give in to stigma; they find ways to push back. For conditions that can be hidden from others, one choice is to conceal them. This is commonly referred to as *passing for normal*. Many people with mild mental illness use this strategy, deciding not to share a diagnosis of anxiety or depression with colleagues or family.

For traits that can't be masked, like body weight or physical disabilities, people have fewer options. Sometimes they withdraw socially. Sometimes they fight the stereotypes that reinforce the stigma, such as protecting how hard they work or how capable they are. Sometimes they work to change the story around their attribute. For example, parents may pursue a diagnosis of ADHD for their children to prove that the "bad" behavior is not the result of poor parenting. E-cigarette users often explain their use of nicotine through vaping as safer than traditional smoking, thereby pushing for more acceptability.[14]

Finding supportive allies who are dealing with the same stigma or "wise others" who understand and can sympathize also helps many deal with stigma, as we discussed in the last chapter. It can also provide people with a sense of belonging and boost self-esteem and psychological resilience to the effects of stigma. For example, older deaf people in California have been found to identify as members of a supportive community. These meaningful social connections to others helps them to manage stigma as they age and navigate disability. Similarly, women in Ontario living with HIV have rallied together through friendships, support groups, and church membership to resist self-blame.[15]

Joining together with like-minded others can also create political opportunities to challenge the structural basis of stigma, such as through public protest. When the ACT UP AIDS activist movement started in New York and San Francisco in the late 1980s, half of all Americans wanted people with HIV quarantined. Through "die-ins" and other public displays of collective outrage, they successfully pushed for major investments in HIV research and drug trials. Their tactics were shocking at the time. They invaded medical presentations wearing lab coats, and they chanted *"Fight back! Fight AIDS!"* at baseball games. They disrupted television productions portraying people with HIV as purposeful killers, and they wore shirts stained with bloody handprints to show they were victims of government power.[16] But, as we discussed in chapter 7, this was an incredibly effective and successful approach.

5. Stigma has power that can be harnessed.

Power relations are central to the *perpetuation* of stigma. By *power*, we mean the ability to maintain your own interests and get what you want or need.[17] Power makes it possible for members of one group to stigmatize members of another group.

Because stigma creates barriers to some groups getting resources, it can be a tool for reinforcing authority and privilege and can be mobilized to maintain the social order.[18] The disparaging ways people talk about specific urban neighborhoods, which we discussed in chapter 9, is a good example of this. When neighborhoods are already characterized by low income, minority status, and other stigmatized traits, this facilitates political processes that deny further amenities. The neighborhoods then end up with more underfunded schools, more polluting industries, and more intensive policing.

The story of Hawai'i in chapter 3 is an excellent historical example of the power relations that drive stigma. Leprosy stigma was used to legitimize the types of exclusions and discriminations that kept others down, to reinforce the advantaged position and authority of the Anglo-American elite. Accordingly, academic definitions of stigma are evolving to emphasize that it can only persist in a context where those in power *allow* it to do so.[19]

6. Stigma is self-reinforcing.

One reason that stigmas reinforce low power so effectively is that they tend to cluster and layer together (e.g., HIV, tuberculosis, homelessness, and drug addiction). This compounding of stigma can be exacerbated by other co-occurring structural vulnerabilities such as poverty, sexism, and racism. The intersectional clustering of other stigmas and diseases can act at the same time to *legitimize* the stigmatized nature of each.

The case of neighborhood stigma in Phoenix that we discussed in chapter 9 is also a good example of this clustering. Many people living in the most stigmatized neighborhoods are dealing with the stress of undocumented immigration and the threat of deportation. They are unable to get steady paid work, lack health insurance coverage, and may not be able to get enough to eat. They have higher risk of obesity, diabetes, depression, tuberculosis, asthma, and many other infectious diseases and conditions compared to other areas of the city. The compounding of all these stigmas then further denies them access to the types of political, social, and economic resources with which they might otherwise be able to improve their living conditions or challenge the social order.[20]

The implications of this is that compounding, reinforcing stigmas are much harder to intervene on and improve than simplistic stigmas. Furthermore, people suffering from such stigmas are much more vulnerable and should be treated with greater sensitivity by health and medical professionals.

7. Stigma may confer other benefits.

The points above suggest that stigma persists within complex, hierarchical societies because it allows some people to maintain and grow their power over others. Yet, as we discuss in chapter 8 on mental illness, stigma is also apparent in smaller, more egalitarian societies. So why would stigma exist where there is no clear power advantage? Put another way, why would a species that relies heavily on culture and cooperation have a universal capacity to so readily reject its own?

In applying evolutionary theory, some social scientists explain stigma as an evolved cognitive mechanism. It helps avoid some of the major inherent pitfalls of being an ultra-social species.[21] People, it seems, can only manage a finite number of relationships.[22] Thus, having a means to easily discriminate who might be the best people with whom to engage in trade or other social exchanges (having sex, getting married, making friends) makes sense. It makes those who do the stigmatizing of others feel closer to and identify more with each other. It can help reinforce in-group membership and provide social cohesion.

Another theory, also difficult to test directly, is that the human capacity to stigmatize is a protective mechanism that helps humans actively avoid contagion. This would fit with some scholars' reports that the types of stigmas most commonly seen in small-scale societies relate to hygiene or symptoms of possible parasitic disease, like skin lesions. It also makes sense in light of the observation, discussed in chapter 2, that there is a clear propensity for people to react to most stigmatized traits as if they are contagious—with emotions like disgust, anger and fear—even when they rationally understand that the traits are not *really* dangerous at all and don't in fact associate them with disease.

These two theories explain an obvious contradiction in the current academic scholarship on stigma as it relates to global health. Political-economic analyses, which focus on how "stigma power" is produced and reinforced structurally, show how stigma can be deployed to block access to basic resources like food, water, and healthcare. This then leads to self-fulfilling and often deadly cycles of illness that reinforce the existing power structure. In this view, *global health efforts* are the *solution* to the problem of stigma. They break the cycle of need and allow people to thrive.

On the other hand, evolutionary models highlight the connection between the human tendency to create social and physical distance from things deemed disgusting, improper, or undesirable and the need for adaptive strategies to avoid contagion in our hypersocial species. In this approach, *stigma* is the *solution* to the problem of global health. This helps explain why stigma exists and persists even when there seems nothing ostensibly to be gained, no "stigma power."

The two models are not, actually, incompatible. An evolved mechanism that aided survival and reproduction in the deep human past could easily be exploited for power as societies grow more complex and inequalities begin to emerge. However, the academic scholarship has done little to integrate these two perspectives. Clearly, the field needs better, deeper theoretical synthesis to understand stigma in the context of global public health before we can develop any sort of comprehensive strategy to fix it.

8. Stigma is a major underlying driver of global disease.

As this entire book illustrates, stigma sickens and kills. First, anticipating or experiencing stigma changes people's health-seeking decisions and narrows their options. To avoid humiliation, people deny the signs of illness or avoid medical treatment. Sexually transmitted diseases like syphilis and gonorrhea are highly contagious, but most are easily treatable once diagnosed. However, people avoid treatment or telling their partners about their condition because they fear being labeled as promiscuous. Stigma also drives us to disconnect from a whole host of opportunities and efforts around us that could help. It creates a "why bother?" mentality.[23] As a result, epidemics spread even faster.

Second, being discriminated against, socially rejected, treated unfairly, and feeling low on the social hierarchy are physiologically stressful.[24] Humiliation and shame, the emotions that stigma promotes, are especially intensely felt. Rooted in the mammalian fight-or-flight response, the body adaptively and instinctively reacts. It raises blood pressure, hormone cortisol levels, and pro-inflammatory cytokines. Prolonged, chronic activation of these stress-response systems can lead to impaired immune function, making illness more likely. If this happens chronically, it can accelerate a variety of negative conditions such as cardiovascular disease, unwanted weight gain, and diabetes, as discussed in chapter 6. Moreover, as we also discussed at length in chapter 9, because stigma erodes our most intimate sense of self and identity, and, in so doing, drives mental illness, too.

Third, stigma that is enacted as systematic and systemic discrimination means less access to all the resources that are needed to help us stay well. Concretely, these are basic things like food, water, healthcare, and steady employment. Equally important, stigma prevents us from accessing social support and feeling we have value in the world.

Finally, as explained through the cases of depression and obesity, stigmas and other vulnerabilities such as poverty and lack of political power tend to clump together, and hence compound the illness and suffering of each. Anthropologists have termed these powerful, complicated, often locked-in, processes stigma syndemics.[25] Together, as we showed in chapter 6 in relation to the example of obesity, these add up to a growing set of reasons we need to start studying stigma as a major driver of global health disparities.

Notes

Introduction. Why We Wrote This Book

1. "Emma" was interviewed as part of a study in the southeastern United States. Elizabeth A. Rohan, Jennifer Boehm, Kristine Gabuten Allen, and Jon Poehlman, "In Their Own Words: A Qualitative Study of the Psychosocial Concerns of Posttreatment and Long-Term Lung Cancer Survivors," *Journal of Psychosocial Oncology* 34, no. 3 (2016): 169–183.

2. The appendix provides a primer of current academic understandings of stigma as related to health. The best general academic book explaining the notion of stigma more generally remains the first: Erving Goffman, *Stigma: Notes of the Management of Spoiled Identity* (New York: Simon and Shuster, 1963). Other more recent recommended syntheses of the academic literature are Bernice A. Pescosolido, Jack K. Martin, Annie Lang, and Sigrun Olafsdottir, "Rethinking Theoretical Approaches to Stigma: A Framework Integrating Normative Influences on Stigma (FINIS)," *Social Science & Medicine* 67 (2008): 431–440; Brenda Major and Laurie T. O'Brien, "The Social Psychology of Stigma," *Annual Review of Psychology* 56 (2005): 393–421; Lawrence Yang, Arthur Kleinman, Bruce G. Link, Jo C. Phelan, Sing Lee, and Byron Good, "Culture and Stigma: Adding Moral Experience to Stigma Theory," *Social Science & Medicine* 64 (2007): 1524–1535; Bruce G. Link and Jo C. Phelan, "Conceptualizing Stigma," *Annual Review of Sociology* 27 (2001): 363–385; Mark L. Hatzenbuehler, Jo C. Phelan, and Bruce G. Link, "Stigma as a Fundamental Cause of Population Health Inequalities," *American Journal of Public Health* 103 (2012): 813–821.

3. For a detailed discussion, see Ronald Bayer and Jennifer Stuber, "Tobacco Control, Stigma, and Public Health: Rethinking the Relations," *American Journal of Public Health* 96 (2006): 47–50.

4. This notion of "exiles among the healthy" is taken from Anne Grethe Halding, Kristin Heggdal, and Astrid Wahl, "Experiences of Self-Blame and Stigmatisation for Self-Infliction among Individuals Living with COPD," *Scandinavian Journal of Caring Sciences* 25 (2011): 100–107.

5. James Zabora, Karlynn BrintzenhofeSzoc, Barbara Curbow, Craig Hooker, and Steven Piantadosi, "The Prevalence of Psychological Distress by Cancer Site," *Psycho-Oncology* 10, no. 1 (2001): 19–28.

6. The tobacco companies also moved aggressively to create new markets in middle- and lower-income countries, and now this is where nearly 80 percent of all smokers live. Many spend a large percentage of otherwise small incomes on tobacco.

7. Recently, other scholars have reacted with similar concern around the issues of shame in CLTS. Myles Bateman and Susan Engel, "To Shame or Not to Shame—That Is the Sanitation Question," *Development Policy Review* 36, no. 2 (2018): 155–173.

8. The 1997 book by journalist Randy Shilts, *And the Band Played On* (St. Martin's Press), describes in detail how this played out in the United States.

9. Rajalakshmi Lakshman, David Ogilvie, and Ken Ong, "Mothers' Experiences of Bottle Feeding: A Systematic Review of Qualitative and Quantitative Studies," *Archives of Disease in Childhood* 94, no. 8 (2009): 596.

10. See, for example, Lyla Mehta and Synne Movik, eds., *Shit Matters: The Potential of Community-Led Total Sanitation* (Bourton-on-Dunsmore, UK: Practical Action Publishing, 2011). Mary Galvin, "Talking Shit: Is Community-Led Total Sanitation a Radical and Revolutionary Approach to Sanitation?" *Wiley Interdisciplinary Reviews* 2, no. 1 (2015): 9–20.

11. An excellent review and exposition on this is Hatzenbuehler, Phelan, Link, "Stigma as a Fundamental Cause," 813–821.

12. Lawrence H. Yang, Fang-pei Chen, Kathleen Janel Sia, Jonathan Lam, Katherine Lam, Hong Ngo, Sing Lee, Arthur Kleinman, and Byron Good, "What Matters Most: A Cultural Mechanism Moderating Structural Vulnerability and Moral Experience of Mental Illness Stigma," *Social Science & Medicine* 103 (2014): 84–93.

13. Here we are distinguishing between "disease" as an actual organic dysfunction, such as caused by a virus, representing what the patient has, and "illness" as what the patient feels, the subjective experience of suffering. Whereas disease is something that happens to an individual body, the experience of illness often extends to the family and connected others who struggling to understand and treat the disease. See Cecil G. Helman, "Disease Versus Illness in General Practice," *The Journal of the Royal College of General Practitioners* 31, no. 230 (1981): 548–552; Arthur Kleinman, Leon Eisenberg, and Byron Good, "Culture, Illness, and Care: Clinical Lessons from Anthropologic and Cross-Cultural Research," *Annals of Internal Medicine* 88, no. 2 (1978): 251–258.

14. By "ethnography" here, we mean the writing in detail about cultural and social phenomena based on insights derived from systematic collection and (usually inductive) analysis of field-based data collection through participant observation, done in the field and in communities with which the ethnographer has gained long-term familiarity. While methods of ethnography are applied across many fields, the very detailed forms of case study ethnography we refer to here are written by anthropologists.

15. Paul Farmer, *AIDS and Accusation: Haiti and the Geography of Blame* (Berkeley: University of California Press, 1992); João Biehl, *Vita: Life in a Zone of Social Abandonment* (Berkeley: University of California Press, 2005); Joan Ablon, *Little People in America: The Social Dimensions of Dwarfism* (New York: Praeger Publishing, 1984); Cassandra White, *An Uncertain Cure: Living with Leprosy in Brazil* (Studies in Medical Anthropology) (New Brunswick: Rutgers University Press, 2009); Marcia C. Inhorn, *Quest for Conception: Gender, Infertility and Egyptian Medical Traditions* (Philadelphia: University of Pennsylvania Press, 1994); Charles L. Briggs, *Stories in the Time of Cholera: Racial Profiling during a Medical Nightmare* (Berkeley: University of California Press, 2003).

16. Erving Goffman, while he identified as a sociologist through much of his career, did much of his seminal academic work on stigma using the tools of detailed ethnography. See Erving Goffman, *Asylums: Essays on the Social Situation of Mental Patients and Other Inmates* (England: Penguin, 1961); Erving Goffman, "The Presentation of Self in Everyday Life," *American Journal of Sociology* 55 (1949): 6–7. The latter was based on his PhD dissertation. *Asylums* got real attention and spurred some change around abuses in mental health treatment. Even so, stigma was slow to change in mental health treatment circles.

17. Obvious exceptions within anthropology include work on syndemics, structural violence, and moral worlds. See, for example, Merill Singer and Scott Clair, "Syndemics and Public Health: Reconceptualizing Disease in Bio-Social Context," *Medical Anthropology Quarterly* 17, no. 4 (2003): 423–441; Arachu Castro and Paul Farmer, "Understanding and Addressing AIDS-Related Stigma: From Anthropological Theory to Clinical Practice in Haiti," *American Journal of Public Health* 95, no. 1 (2005): 53–59; Yang, Kleinman, Link, Phelan, Lee, Good, "Culture and Stigma," 1524–1535.

18. Much of our field-based research is based on a strategy of creating knowledge through systematic comparison of cultural data across diverse sites. For example, Alexandra Brewis, Asher Rosinger, Amber Wutich, Ellis Adams, Lee Cronk, Amber Pearson, Cassandra Workman, Sera Young, and the HWISE Consortium, "Water Sharing, Reciprocity, and Need: A Comparative Study of Inter-Household Water Transfers in Sub-Saharan Africa," *Economic Anthropology* 6, no. 2 (2019): 208–211, https://doi.org/10.1002/sea2.12143; Amber Wutich, Alexandra Brewis, Abigail M. York, and Rhian Stotts, "Rules, Norms, and Injustice: A Cross-Cultural Study of Perceptions of Justice in Water Institutions," *Society & Natural Resources* 26, no. 7 (2013): 795–809; Alexandra A. Brewis, Meredith Gartin, Amber Wutich, and Alyson Young, "Global Convergence in Ethnotheories of Water and Disease," *Global Public Health* 8, no. 1 (2013): 13–36; Alexandra A. Brewis, Amber Wutich, Ashlan Falletta-Cowden, and Isa Rodriguez-Soto, "Body Norms and Fat Stigma in Global Perspective," *Current Anthropology* 52, no. 2 (2011): 269–276; Cindi SturtzSreetharan, Alexandra Brewis, Monet Niesluchowski, and Amber Wutich, "'Do I look fat?' The Global Form of Women's Fat Talk" (forthcoming).

19. For details on cutting-edge approaches to systematic qualitative research see H. Russell Bernard, Amber Wutich, and Gery W. Ryan, *Analyzing Qualitative Data: Systematic Approaches* (Thousand Oaks, CA: SAGE Publications, 2016).

20. For example, Saul D. Alinsky, "The War on Poverty-Political Pornography," *Journal of Social Issues* 21, no. 1 (1965): 41–47; D. Goldfinger, "Development Pornography: Images of the Global South," *Artishake* 2 (2006): 4–5.

21. By "power," we mean the capacity to get what you want, socially, politically, and economically. Wealth is one easily deployed form of power.

22. Noting that part of this success was in showing different, "blame-free" faces of the disease. American Ryan White died of AIDS in 1990 at the age of eighteen. His case profoundly changed public attitudes toward HIV/AIDS because he was seen as a completely blameless victim of what—prior to that time—was seen as a disease of people who made serious lifestyle mistakes. Born with hemophilia, he contracted HIV through his life-saving blood transfusions. Once infected with HIV,

he was rejected by his school and classmates. A difficult legal battle followed. He spoke publicly—and very well—and gathered the support of many celebrities. His case spurred significant change in public fear toward HIV/AIDS. The 1990 Ryan White CARE Act voted more than $2 billion for better community-based prevention, diagnosis, and care around HIV in the United States.

23. A "wicked problem" is diabolically difficult to solve because it is contradictory, confusing, tricky to recognize, and hard to define with any precision.

Chapter 1. Dealing with Defecation

1. United Nations International Children's Emergency Fund, *UNICEF Current Situation in Mozambique*, http://www.unicef.org.mz/en/our-work/what-we-do/water -sanitation-hygiene/; Annette Prüss, David Kay, Lorna Fewtrell, and Jamie Bartram, "Estimating the Burden of Disease from Water, Sanitation, and Hygiene at a Global Level," *Environmental Health Perspectives* 110, no. 5 (2002): 537–542; "Mozambique," Community-Led Total Sanitation, http://www .communityledtotalsanitation.org/country/mozambique; Deise I. Galan, Seung-Sup Kim, and Jay P. Graham, "Exploring Changes in Open Defecation Prevalence in sub-Saharan Africa Based on National Level Indices," *BMC Public Health* 13, no. 1 (2013): 527. People are often reticent to speak to interviewers about their toileting habits. The rates are probably much higher.

2. The initial survey of 1,226 households in neighborhoods of low, medium, and higher flood risk was conducted in Pemba in July 2016, as part of the baseline of the USAID-funded Coastal Cities Adaptation Project (CCAP). A follow-up interview with 212 households, reselected using the same geographic sampling strategy, yielded the same result (~10–12 percent non-use of toilets).

3. The average human produces around 128 gm/day of feces. C. Rose, Alison Parker, Bruce Jefferson, and Elise Cartmell, "The Characterization of Feces and Urine: A Review of the Literature to Inform Advanced Treatment Technology," *Critical Reviews in Environmental Science and Technology* 45, no. 17 (2015): 1827–1879. The domesticated animals and pets that we share our lives with add to our daily contact with fecal contaminants. Kay Prüss and Bartram Fewtrell, "Estimating the Burden of Disease from Water, Sanitation, and Hygiene at the Global Level," *Environmental Health Perspectives* 110, no. 5 (2002): 537–542.

4. "Improved sanitation" refers to facilities that hygienically separate human excreta from human contact, such as a flushing or composting toilet.

5. Tacilta Nhampossa, Inacio Mandomando, Sozinho Acacio, Llorenç Quintó, Delfino Vubil, Joaquin Ruiz, Delino Nhalungo, et al., "Diarrheal Disease in Rural Mozambique: Burden, Risk Factors and Etiology of Diarrheal Disease among Children Aged 0–59 Months Seeking Care at Health Facilities," *PloS One* 10, no. 5 (2015): e0119824; Kay Prüss and Bartram Fewtrell, "Estimating the Burden of Disease," 537–542; Valerie Curtis, Wolf Schmidt, Stephen Luby, Rocio Florez, Ousmane Touré, and Adam Biran, "Hygiene: New Hopes, New Horizons," *The Lancet Infectious Diseases* 11, no. 4 (2011): 312–321; Valerie Curtis and Sandy Cairncross, "Effect of Washing Hands with Soap on Diarrhoea Risk in the Community: A Systematic Review," *The Lancet Infectious Diseases* 3, no. 5 (2003): 275–281.

6. Curtis, Schmidt, Luby, Florez, Touré, and Biran, "Hygiene: New Hopes," 312–321; Curtis and Cairncross, "Effect of Washing Hands," 275–281.

7. G. D. Sclar, G. Penakalapati, B. A. Caruso, Eva Annette Rehfuess, J. V. Garn, K. T. Alexander, M. C. Freeman, S. Boisson, K. Medlicott, and T. Clasen, "Exploring the relationship between sanitation and mental and social well-being: A systematic review and qualitative synthesis," *Social Science & Medicine* 217 (2018): 121–134. For examples from India: Vijay Raju, "To Achieve Gender Equality in India, Build More Toilets," World Economic Forum, https://www.weforum.org /agenda/2016/10/to-achieve-gender-equality-build-more-toilets; Seema Kulkarni, Kathleen O'Reilly, and Sneha Bhat, "No relief: Lived Experiences of Inadequate Sanitation Access of Poor Urban Women in India," *Gender & Development* 25, no. 2 (2017): 167–183.

8. The late anthropologist Ward H. Goodenough penned a delightful essay on his experiences using an overwater latrine in Kiribati. Philip R. DeVita, *The Humbled Anthropologist: Tales from the Pacific* (Nashville: Wadsworth, 1990).

9. Pauline A. Jumaa, "Hand Hygiene: Simple and Complex," *International Journal of Infectious Diseases* 9, no. 1 (2005): 3–14; Matthew C. Freeman, Meredith E. Stocks, Oliver Cumming, Aurelie Jeandron, Julian P. T. Higgins, Jennyfer Wolf, Annette Prüss-Ustün, Sophie Bonjour, Paul R. Hunter, Lorna Fewtrell, and Valerie Curtis, "Systematic Review: Hygiene and Health: Systematic Review of Handwashing Practices Worldwide and Update of Health Effects," *Tropical Medicine & International Health* 19, no. 8 (2014): 906–916. Global rates of handwashing with soap are reportedly highest in New Zealand and lowest in Tanzania. In no country does it exceed 60 percent.

10. Jacqueline Randle, Antony Kobina Arthur, and Natalie Vaughan, "Twenty-Four-Hour Observational Study of Hospital Hand Hygiene Compliance," *Journal of Hospital Infection* 76, no. 3 (2010): 252–255.

11. Bruno Cardinale Lagomarsino, Matías Gutman, Lucía Freira, María Laura Lanzalot, Maximiliano Lauletta, Leandro E. Malchik, Felipe Montaño Campos, Bianca Pacini, Martín A. Rossi, and Christian Valencia, "Peer Pressure: Experimental Evidence from Restroom Behavior," *Economic Inquiry* 55, no. 3 (2017): 1579–1584.

12. This is a shared global goal for development, enacted through global health. The United Nations Sustainable Development Goal (SDG) 6.2 aims to "achieve access to adequate and equitable sanitation and hygiene for all and end open defecation." UN-Water, http://www.sdg6monitoring.org/indicators/target-6-2/. Even as rates are declining, open defecation remains extremely common in many lower-income countries, especially in Asia and sub-Saharan Africa. Numerically, India has the highest number of people without access to a toilet at over 500 million; globally the number is over 2 billion and many of these are living in rural areas. World Health Organization (WHO) and the United Nations Children's Fund (UNICEF), *Progress on Drinking Water, Sanitation and Hygiene: 2017 Update and SDG Baselines* (Geneva: World Health Organization, 2017).

13. United Nations International Children's Emergency Fund, "Evaluation of the WASH Sector Strategy 'Community Approaches to Total Sanitation' (CATS) Final Evaluation Report," UNICEF.org, https://www.unicef.org/evaldatabase/files /Final_Evaluation_Report_CATS.pdf.

14. Duncan Mara, Jon Lane, Beth Scott, and David Trouba, "Sanitation and Health," *PLoS Medicine* 7, no. 11 (2010): e1000363.

15. United Nations International Children's Emergency Fund, "Evaluation of the Wash." Gaby Judah, Robert Aunger, Wolf-Peter Schmidt, Susan Michie, Stewart Granger, and Val Curtis, "Experimental Pretesting of Hand-Washing Interventions in a Natural Setting," *American Journal of Public Health* 99, no. S2 (2009): S405–S411; Renata Porzig-Drummond, Richard Stevenson, Trevor Case, and Megan Oaten, "Can the Emotion of Disgust be Harnessed to Promote Hand Hygiene? Experimental and Field-Based Tests," *Social Science & Medicine* 68, no. 6 (2009): 1006–1012; Beth E. Scott, Wolf P. Schmidt, Robert Aunger, Nana Garbrah-Aidoo, and Rasaaque Animashaun, "Marketing Hygiene Behaviours: The Impact of Different Communication Channels on Reported Handwashing Behaviour of Women in Ghana," *Health Education Research* 23, no. 3 (2007): 392–401.

16. United Nations International Children's Emergency Fund, "'Community Led Total Sanitation' Initiative," UNICEF.org, https://www.unicef.org/wash /mozambique_53709.html.

17. "Mozambique," Community-Led Total Sanitation, http://www .communityledtotalsanitation.org/country/mozambique.

18. United Nations International Children's Emergency Fund, "Evaluation of the Wash."

19. Using behavior-centered design for the SuperAmma campaign resulted in observations of increased handwashing, with disgust, status, affiliation, and fear deployed as its key motivators. SuperAmma, "SuperAmma Campaign for Changing Hand Washing Behaviour," superamma.org, http://www.superamma .org; Adam Biran, Wolf-Peter Schmidt, Kiruba Sankar Varadharajan, Divya Rajaraman, Raja Kumar, Katie Greenland, Balaji Gopalan, Robert Aunger, and Val Curtis, "Effect of a Behaviour-Change Intervention on Handwashing with Soap in India (SuperAmma): A Cluster-Randomised Trial," *The Lancet Global Health* 2, no. 3 (2014): e145–e154.

20. Valerie A. Curtis, Lisa O. Danquah, and Robert V. Aunger, "Planned, Motivated and Habitual Hygiene Behaviour: An Eleven Country Review," *Health Education Research* 24, no. 4 (2009): 655–673.

21. Amy J. Pickering, Habiba Djebbari, Carolina Lopez, Massa Coulibaly, and Maria Laura Alzua, "Effect of a Community-Led Sanitation Intervention on Child Diarrhoea and Child Growth in Rural Mali: A Cluster-Randomised Controlled Trial," *The Lancet Global Health* 3, no. 11 (2015): e701–e711.

22. SuperAmma, "SuperAmma Campaign."

23. United Nations International Children's Emergency Fund, "Evaluation of the WASH." Rachel Sigler, Lyana Mahmoudi, and Jay Paul Graham, "Analysis of Behavioral Change Techniques in Community-Led Total Sanitation Programs," *Health Promotion International* 30, no. 1 (2014): 16–28.

24. Paul Ekman, "Are There Basic Emotions?" *Psychological Review* 99, no. 3 (1992): 550–553; Paul Ekman, "An Argument for Basic Emotions," *Cognition and Emotion* 6, no. 3: 169–200; Paul Rozin, Laura Lowery, and Rhonda Ebert, "Varieties of Disgust Faces and the Structure of Disgust," *Journal of Personality and Social Psychology* 66, no. 5 (1994): 870; Charles Darwin, with Paul Ekman and Phillip Prodger, *The Expression of the Emotions in Man and Animals* (London: HarperCollins, 1998).

25. Ekman, "An Argument," 169–200; Randolph M. Nesse and George C. Williams, *Why We Get Sick: The New Science of Darwinian Medicine* (New York:

Vintage Books, 2012); M. L. Phillips, C. Senior, T. Fahy, and A. S. David, "Disgust—The Forgotten Emotion of Psychiatry," *The British Journal of Psychiatry* 172, no. 5 (1998): 373–375; Sandy Cairncross, "Handwashing With Soap—A New Way to Prevent ARIs?" *Tropical Medicine & International Health* 8, no. 8 (2003): 677–679; Sarah Wilson, Casey J. Jacob, and Douglas Powell, "Behavior-Change Interventions to Improve Hand-Hygiene Practice: A Review of Alternatives to Education," *Critical Public Health* 21, no. 1 (2011): 119–127.

26. John S. Allen, *The Omnivorous Mind: Our Evolving Relationship with Food* (Cambridge, MA: Harvard University Press, 2012). Allen explains this argument in detail regarding why basic disgust reactions are so key to our species' survival.

27. Steven L. Neuberg, Dylan M. Smith, and Terrilee Asher, "Why People Stigmatize: Toward a Biocultural Framework," in *The Social Psychology of Stigma* (New York: Guilford Press, 2000), 31–61; Steven L. Neuberg, Douglas T. Kenrick, and Mark Schaller, "Human Threat Management Systems: Self-Protection and Disease Avoidance," *Neuroscience & Biobehavioral Reviews* 35, no. 4 (2011): 1042–1051; Robert Kurzban and Mark R. Leary, "Evolutionary Origins of Stigmatization: The Functions of Social Exclusion," *Psychological Bulletin* 127, no. 2 (2001): 187; Liz Chatterjee, "Time to Acknowledge the Dirty Truth Behind Community-Led Sanitation," *The Guardian*, June 9, 2011, https://www.theguardian.com/global -development/poverty-matters/2011/jun/09/dirty-truth-behind-community -sanitation; Megan Oaten, Richard J. Stevenson, and Trevor I. Case, "Disease Avoidance as a Functional Basis for Stigmatization," *Philosophical Transactions of the Royal Society of London B: Biological Sciences* 366, no. 1583 (2011): 3433–3452. Evolutionarily oriented social scientists explain stigma as an evolved cognitive mechanism that helps avoid some of the major inherent pitfalls of being an ultra-social species. Some suggest that people can only manage a finite number of relationships, so having a means to easily discriminate who might be the best people with whom to engage in trade or other social exchanges (having sex, getting married) makes sense. Leary Kurzban, "Evolutionary Origins," 187. Stigmatizing and otherwise defining outsiders by any means can also help promote potentially advantageous in-group social cohesion. Carlos David Navarrete and Daniel M. T. Fessler, "Disease Avoidance and Ethnocentrism: The Effects of Disease Vulnerability and Disgust Sensitivity on Intergroup Attitudes," *Evolution and Human Behavior* 27, no. 4 (2006): 270–282.

28. Fistulas can also be caused by the physical trauma of rape.

29. L. Lewis Wall, *Tears for My Sisters: The Tragedy of Obstetric Fistula* (Baltimore: Johns Hopkins University Press, 2018).

30. Even development and health workers trying to help fistula-affected women can be overcome by pity. They dismiss them as "poor little girls," "the wretched of the earth," and even "women who cannot even be successful prostitutes." Maggie Bangser, "Obstetric Fistula and Stigma," *The Lancet* 367, no. 9509 (2006): 535–536; Janet Molzan Turan, Khaliah Johnson, and Mary Lake Polan, "Experiences of Women Seeking Medical Care for Obstetric Fistula in Eritrea: Implications for Prevention, Treatment, and Social Reintegration," *Global Public Health* 2, no. 1 (2007): 64–77.

31. Exactly what people identify as morally disgusting does vary culturally. Americans say they are disgusted by those who abandon their elderly parents and,

increasingly, by those on the other side of political divides. But the greatest moral disgust expressed by Americans stems from gross violations of human bodies and dignity like rape, murder, and child abuse. By contrast, Japanese disgust reactions (*ken'o*) are more tied to small, everyday events—things like being shamed for driving poorly or failing an exam. That is, stigma is about the shame of not being the person you *should* be. See Mark Schaller, Damian R. Murray, and Adrian Bangerter, "Implications of the Behavioural Immune System for Social Behaviour and Human Health in the Modern World," *Philosophical Transactions of the Royal Society of London B: Biological Sciences*, no. 1669 (2015): 20140105.

32. Thomas Buckley and Alma Gottlieb, eds., *Blood Magic: The Anthropology of Menstruation* (Berkeley: University of California Press, 1988).

33. The practice of *chhaupadi*, this type of menstrual segregation, is illegal but persists. Mary Crawford, Lauren M. Menger, and Michelle R. Kaufman, "'This is a Natural Process': Managing Menstrual Stigma in Nepal," *Culture, Health & Sexuality* 16, no. 4 (2014): 426–439.

34. Chhabi Ranabhat, Chun-Bae Kim, Eun Hee Choi, Anu Aryal, Myung Bae Park, and Young Ah Doh, "Chhaupadi Culture and Reproductive Health of Women in Nepal," *Asia Pacific Journal of Public Health* 27, no. 7 (2015): 785–795.

35. Danielle Preiss, "A Young Woman Died in A Menstrual Hut in Nepal," NPR .org, https://www.npr.org/sections/goatsandsoda/2016/11/28/503155803/a -young-woman-died-in-a-menstrual-shed-in-nepal.

36. Similarly, a man with a sexually transmitted disease like herpes or chlamydia might be judged as a player or sexual conqueror. A woman with the same disease is more likely to be judged as promiscuous.

37. UNICEF, "Community-led Total Sanitation in East Asia and Pacific: Progress, Lessons and Directions" (Bangkok: UNICEF, 2013).

38. "Kiribati," Community-Led Total Sanitation, http://www .communityledtotalsanitation.org/country/kiribati.

39. At least some sanitation experts have sensibly suggested the need to avoid shaming if at all possible. "WaterAid Hygiene Framework," wateraid.org. www .wateraid.org/publications. Mary Galvin, "Talking Shit: Is Community-Led Total Sanitation a Radical and Revolutionary Approach to Sanitation?" *Wiley Interdisciplinary Reviews: Water* 2, no. 1 (2015): 9–20; Margaret C. Morales, and Leila M. Harris, "Using Subjectivity and Emotion to Reconsider Participatory Natural Resource Management," *World Development* 64 (2014): 703–712; Sameer Sah and Amsalu Negussie, "Community Led Total Sanitation (CLTS): Addressing the Challenges of Scale and Sustainability in Rural Africa," *Desalination* 248, no. 1–3 (2009): 666–672.

40. Amina Mahbub, "Social Dynamics of CLTS: Inclusion of Children, Women and Vulnerable," In *CLTS Conference* (2008): 16–18.

41. Galvin points out this isn't so strange. Even many highly educated, urban people don't use seatbelts, smoke, and eat fatty food to excess. Long-term behavior changes around things that have deep meaning, are addictive, or just feel really good—even when highly motivated—is really hard; Mary Galvin, "Talking Shit: Is Community-Led Total Sanitation a Radical and Revolutionary Approach to Sanitation?" *Wiley Interdisciplinary Reviews: Water* 2, no. 1 (2015): 9–20.

42. Based on online surveys of staff who implemented community-based sanitation programs, only 8 percent of respondents mentioned negative

outcomes. The nature of the negative outcomes was not reported. "WaterAid," wateraid.org.

43. Peter A. Harvey, "Zero Subsidy Strategies for Accelerating Access to Rural Water and Sanitation Services," *Water Science and Technology* 63, no. 5 (2011): 1037–1043.

44. For example, Kathleen O'Reilly, Richa Dhanju, and Elizabeth Louis, "Subjected to Sanitation: Caste Relations and Sanitation Adoption in Rural Tamil Nadu," *The Journal of Development Studies* 53, no. 11 (2017): 1915–1928. In another ethnographically oriented study in Zambia, women felt they were expected to press their husbands to build latrines. But they worried this "nagging" distracted in damaging ways from other family needs they felt obliged to attend to (like money for schooling). Those without social networks—often those otherwise most burdened already by widowhood, age, poverty, or illness—struggled most to meet the village expectations of complete open-defecation-free status. Kevin, Bardosh, "Achieving 'Total Sanitation' in Rural African Geographies: Poverty, Participation and Pit Latrines in Eastern Zambia," *Geoforum* 66 (2015): 53–63.

45. Lyla Mehta and Synne Movik, eds., *Shit Matters: The Potential of Community-Led Total Sanitation* (Rugby, UK: Practical Action Publishing, 2011).

46. Rachel Sigler, Lyana Mahmoudi, and Jay P. Graham, "Analysis of Behavioral Change Techniques in Community-Led Total Sanitation Programs," *Health Promotion International* 30, no. 1 (2015): 16–28.

47. Jori Lewis, "Ending Open Defecation: A Review of Community-Led Sanitation Programs," *Environmental Health Perspectives* 126, no. 4 (2018), doi: 10.1289/EHP3471.

48. Aashish Gupta, Diane Coffey, and Dean Spears, "Purity, Pollution, and Untouchability: Challenges Affecting the Adoption, Use, and Sustainability of Sanitation Programmes in Rural India," in *Sustainable Sanitation for All: Experiences, Challenges, and Innovations*, ed. P. Bongartz, N. Vernon, and J. Fox (Rugby, UK: Practical Action Publishing, 2016), 283–298; Diane Coffey, Aashish Gupta, Payal Hathi, Dean Spears, Nikhil Srivastav, Sangita Vyas, "Untouchability, Pollution, and Latrine Pits: Understanding Open Defecation in Rural India," *Economic and Political Weekly* 52, no.1 (2017).

49. Julie Watson, Robert Dreibelbis, Robert Aunger, Claudio Deola, Katrice King, Susan Long, Rachel P. Chase, and Oliver Cumming, "Child's Play: Harnessing Play and Curiosity Motives to Improve Child Handwashing in a Humanitarian Setting," *International Journal of Hygiene and Environmental Health* 222, no. 2 (2019): 177–182, doi: 10.1016/j.ijheh.2018.09.002.

50. Mary Galvin, "Talking Shit: Is Community-Led Total Sanitation a Radical and Revolutionary Approach to Sanitation?" *Wiley Interdisciplinary Reviews: Water* 2, no. 1 (2015): 9–20; Jamie Bartram, Katrina Charles, Barbara Evans, Lucinda O'Hanlon, and Steve Pedley, "Commentary on Community-Led Total Sanitation and Human Rights: Should the Right to Community-Wide Health Be Won at the Cost of Individual Rights?" *Journal of Water and Health* 10, no. 4 (2012): 499–503.

Chapter 2. Dirty Things, Disgusting People

1. Mary Douglas, *Purity and Danger: An Analysis of Concepts of Pollution and Taboo* (Abingdon, UK: Routledge, 2003).

2. Andreas De Block and Stefaan E. Cuypers, "Why Darwinians Should Not be Afraid of Mary Douglas—And Vice Versa: The Case of Disgust," *Philosophy of the Social Sciences* 42, no. 4 (2012): 459–488; Megan Oaten, Richard J. Stevenson, and Trevor I. Case, "Disgust as a Disease-Avoidance Mechanism," *Psychological Bulletin* 135, no. 2 (2009): 303; Megan Oaten, Richard J. Stevenson, and Trevor I. Case, "Disease Avoidance as a Functional Basis for Stigmatization," *Philosophical Transactions of the Royal Society of London B: Biological Sciences* 366, no. 1583 (2011): 3433–3452. In the 1980s, previous to this set of research in evolutionary psychology, anthropologist Marvin Harris reanalyzed historical and ethnographic cases to propose that taboos and associated rituals (such as avoidance of pork in Judaism) persisted because they had material functions, such as maintaining safe, sustainable food supplies. Marvin Harris, *Good to Eat: Riddles of Food and Culture* (Long Grove, IL: Waveland Press, 1998).

3. Consider Miner's ethnographic spoof exploring Nicarema (American) obsessive hygiene rituals. Horace Miner, "Body Ritual Among the Nacirema," *American Anthropologist* 58, no. 3 (1956): 503–507. See also Nancy Tomes, *The Gospel of Germs: Men, Women, and the Microbe in American Life* (Cambridge, MA: Harvard University Press, 1999), for a historical perspective on America's obsession with germs.

4. Amber Wutich, Abigail M. York, Alexandra Brewis, Rhian Stotts, and Christopher M. Roberts, "Shared Cultural Norms for Justice in Water Institutions: Results from Fiji, Ecuador, Paraguay, New Zealand, and the US," *Journal of Environmental Management* 113 (2012): 370–76; Kelli L. Larson, Rhian Stotts, Amber Wutich, Alexandra Brewis, and Dave White, "Cross-Cultural Perceptions of Water Risks and Solutions Across Select Sites," *Society & Natural Resources* 29, no. 9 (2016): 1049–1064; Alexandra A. Brewis, Meredith Gartin, Amber Wutich, and Alyson Young, "Global Convergence in Ethnotheories of Water and Disease," *Global Public Health* 8, no. 1 (2013): 13–36; Alissa Ruth, Alexandra Brewis, and Amber Wutich, "The Global Ethnohydrology Study: A Model for Scalable Social Science Intensive Research Experiences," *International Journal of Mass Emergencies and Disasters* (forthcoming).

5. Amber Wutich and Alexandra Brewis, "Primary Data Collection in Cross-cultural Ethnographic Research," *Field Methods* (forthcoming).

6. For example: Brewis, Gartin, Wutich, Young, "Global Convergence," 13–36. Margaret V. Du Bray, Amber Wutich, and Alexandra Brewis, "Hope and Worry: Gendered Emotional Geographies of Climate Change in Three Vulnerable US Communities," *Weather, Climate, and Society* 9, no. 2 (2017): 285–297.

7. Val Curtis, Robert Aunger, and Tamer Rabie, "Evidence that Disgust Evolved to Protect from Risk of Disease," *Proceedings of the Royal Society of London B: Biological Sciences* 271, no. 4 (2004): S131–S133. As part of the procedure, we used "neutral photos" to adjust for community differences in how strong their responses were overall on the Likert-type scales. For example, in New Zealand, people tended to respond with less disgust to both neutral (clean) photos and disgusting ones.

8. For our study, we defined "low waterborne disease risk" as occurring in countries where (1) the percentage of total deaths attributable to water, sanitation, and hygiene was 1 percent or less, and (2) the percentage of deaths of

children under five years of age due to diarrhea was 2 percent or less. We defined sites as having "more water scarcity" if they had either physical water scarcity (as in Arizona, United States) or economic water scarcity (as in Acatenango, Guatemala). For more information on the study, see Alexandra Brewis, Amber Wutich, Megan DuBray, Roseanne Schuster, Jonathan Maupin, and Matthew Gervais, "Community hygiene norm violators are consistently stigmatized: Evidence from four global sites and implications for sanitation interventions," *Social Science and Medicine* 202 (2019): 12–21.

9. Jonathan N. Maupin, "Remaking the Guatemalan Midwife: Health Care Reform and Midwifery Training Programs in Highland Guatemala," *Medical Anthropology* 27, no. 4 (2008): 353–382; Jonathan N. Maupin, "'Fruit of the Accords': Healthcare Reform and Civil Participation in Highland Guatemala," *Social Science & Medicine* 68, no. 8 (2009): 1456–1463; Jonathan N. Maupin, "Divergent Models of Community Health Workers in Highland Guatemala," *Human Organization* (2011): 44–53.

10. Although, after we did this data collection there was a dreadful outbreak of gastrointestinal illness campylobacteriosis in Havelock North in August 2016 that made some four thousand people sick, likely caused by contamination of the water supply with sheep feces.

11. This may be partially explained by a phenomenon known as "social desirability reporting," whereby respondents are swayed by what they think an interviewer wants to hear or is the more socially acceptable answer. It is possible that, in a large city like Phoenix, people cared less about what they admitted to a stranger, especially compared to reporting to a known research team in a small village setting.

12. This was also a surprise finding, especially given that the handwashing literature suggests massive differences in behaviors between Guatemala and New Zealand, for example. It could reflect that people in all the sites are similarly concerned about staying clean and are consistently doing things in their daily lives to meet this goal. Perhaps there would have been more differentiation if we selected communities where resource shortages (e.g., water) were more extreme.

13. Isha Ray, "Women, Water, and Development," *Annual Review of Environment and Resources* 32 (2007); B. Suresh Reddy and M. Snehalatha, "Sanitation and Personal Hygiene: What Does it Mean to Poor and Vulnerable Women?" *Indian Journal of Gender Studies* 18, no. 3 (2011): 381–404; Tina Khanna and Madhumita Das, "Why Gender Matters in the Solution Towards Safe Sanitation? Reflections from Rural India," *Global Public Health* 11, no. 10 (2016): 1185–1201.

14. In addition, there is a large literature on how menstrual taboos and stigma harms women and girls: Amber Wutich and Alexandra Brewis, "Food, Water, and Scarcity: Toward a Broader Anthropology of Resource Insecurity," *Current Anthropology* 55, no. 4 (2014); United Nations Development Programme, *Beyond Scarcity: Power, Poverty and the Global Water Crisis* (New York: Palgrave Macmillan, 2006); Sabina Faiz Rashid and Stephanie Michaud, "Female Adolescents and their Sexuality: Notions of Honour, Shame, Purity and Pollution During the Floods," *Disasters* 24, no. 1 (2000): 54–70.

15. In qualitative and cultural research, it is common for researchers to pick a purposive sample based on intensity—that is, to interview people who researchers

believe will intensely manifest a phenomenon. And that's what we did here. Michael Quinn Patton, *Qualitative Evaluation and Research Methods* (Thousand Oaks, CA: SAGE, 1990) 2, 169–186. Sample sizes were set based on Ashley K. Hagaman and Amber Wutich, "How Many Interviews are Enough to Identify Metathemes in Multisited and Cross-Cultural Research? Another Perspective on Guest, Bunce, and Johnson's (2006) Landmark Study," *Field Methods* 29, no. 1 (2017): 23–41.

16. For an alternative analysis of these hygiene data, see Brewis, Wutich, du Bray, Maupin, Schuster, Gervais, "Community Hygiene Norm Violators."

17. The listed women were selected as typical exemplars for each site, representing common themes at each location. To identify typical exemplars, we used a qualitative method for inter-rater comparison agreement adapted from Ryan (1999) on measuring the typicality of texts. Gery W. Ryan, "Measuring the Typicality of Text: Using Multiple Coders for More Than Just Reliability and Validity Checks," *Human Organization* 58, no. 3 (1999): 313–322.

18. Other respondents in the United States sites concurred, with many also imagining that such a woman would have hair that was "not done" (meaning: inadequately styled) and too little or too much makeup.

19. Anne E. Becker, *Body, Self, and Society: The View from Fiji* (Philadelphia: University of Pennsylvania Press, 1995).

20. New Zealand has recently been identified as having a very high rate of homelessness within the OECD, with more 1 percent of the total population on the streets or in emergency or substandard shelter. University of Otago, "Homelessness Accelerates between Censuses," last modified June 3, 2016, last accessed March 1, 2019, https://www.otago.ac.nz/news/news/otago613529.html.

Chapter 3. Dirty and Disempowered

1. Tonya's story is provided by medical anthropologist Sarah Raskin who interviewed her repeatedly as a key informant during her excellent detailed ethnographic study of dental disease in Appalachia. See Sarah E. Raskin, "Decayed, Missing, and Filled: Subjectivity and the Dental Safety Net in Central Appalachia" (PhD diss., University of Arizona, 2015).

2. "Meth mouth" is proposed to result from some combination of the side effects of methamphetamine use (teeth clenching, dry mouth), lack of preventive care, and a high sugar diet.

3. For example, Jamie Moeller, Sonica Singhal, Mahmoud Al-Dajani, Noha Gomaa, and Carlos Quiñonez, "Assessing the Relationship Between Dental Appearance and the Potential for Discrimination in Ontario, Canada," *SSM-Population Health*, no.1 (2015): 26–31.

4. Mohd Massod, Aubrey Sheiham, and Eduardo Bernabé, "Household Expenditure for Dental Care in Low and Middle Income Countries," *PLoS One* 10, no. 4 (2015): e0123075.

5. L. J. Jin, I. B. Lamster, J. S. Greenspan, N. B. Pitts, C. Scully, and S. Warnakulasuriya, "Global Burden of Oral Diseases: Emerging Concepts, Management and Interplay with Systemic Health," *Oral Diseases* 22, no. 7 (2016): 609–619.

6. Eduardo Bernabé, Mohd Masood, and Marko Vujicic, "The Impact of Out-Of-Pocket Payments for Dental Care on Household Finances in Low and Middle Income Countries," *BMC Public Health* 17, no. 1 (2017): 109.

7. By discrimination, we mean enacted stigma. Things such as being refused jobs or housing, ignored for promotions, or ignored or otherwise mistreated in public spaces like stores or government offices. See this book's appendix for more detailed explanations.

8. Amber interviewed Doña Juana multiple times across 2003–2004 as part of a project studying how the lowest-income urban dwellers cope with chronic water shortages.

9. Renters, new homeowners, and households too poor to pay the required monthly tap stand fee are excluded, and this adds up to nearly three-quarters of residents.

10. Amber Wutich and Kathleen Ragsdale, "Water Insecurity and Emotional Distress: Coping with Supply, Access, and Seasonal Variability of Water in a Bolivian Squatter Settlement," *Social Science & Medicine* 67, no. 12 (2008): 2116–2125; Amber Wutich, "Intrahousehold Disparities in Women and Men's Experiences of Water Insecurity and Emotional Distress in Urban Bolivia," *Medical Anthropology Quarterly* 23, no. 4 (2009): 436–454.

11. Wutich and Ragsdale, "Water Insecurity and Emotional Distress: Coping with Supply, Access, and Seasonal Variability of Water in a Bolivian Squatter Settlement," 2116–2125; Wutich, "Intrahousehold Disparities in Women and Men's Experiences of Water Insecurity and Emotional Distress in Urban Bolivia," 436–454.

12. Some 20 percent of people in developing countries experience clinical levels of depression at some point in their lives. Estimates suggest some 6 percent of men and 10 percent of women globally experience some form of depression in any given year. Most cases probably aren't diagnosed at all either, especially in lower-income nations. See The World Health Report, *Mental Health: New Understanding, New Hope* (Switzerland: World Health Organization, 2001); Alan D. Lopez, Colin D. Mathers, Majid Ezzati, Dean T. Jamison, and Christopher J. L. Murray, "Global and Regional Burden of Disease and Risk Factors, 2001: Systematic Analysis of Population Health Data," *The Lancet* 367, no. 9524 (2006): 1747–1757.

13. Cholera infects the small intestine, causing watery diarrhea and dehydration. With fast treatment, most people survive. But with no or slow treatment, it can cause rapid death. The bacterium is mostly transmitted in drinking water infected by human feces or by eating infected shellfish. See World Health Organization, *Cholera Outbreak: Assessing the Outbreak Response and Improving Preparedness* (Switzerland: World Health Organization, 2004).

14. Santiago Rivera's story was told by medical anthropologists Charles and Clara Briggs. See Charles L. Briggs, and Clara Mantini-Briggs, *Stories in the Time of Cholera: Racial Profiling during a Medical Nightmare* (Berkeley: University of California Press, 2003), 210–211.

15. The story of the Avenida Gonçalves Dias and Dona Zilnar was told by Marilyn K. Nations and Cristina M.G. Monte, "'I'm Not Dog, No!': Cries of Resistance against Cholera Control Campaigns," *Social Science & Medicine* 43, no. 6 (1996): 1007–1024. Quotes are from page 1113. https://doi.org/10.1016/0277 -9536(96)00083-4.

16. Fabini D. Orata, Paul S. Keim, and Yan Boucher, "The 2010 Cholera Outbreak in Haiti: How Science Solved a Controversy," *PLoS Pathogens* 10, no. 4

(2014): e1003967; F. Houghton, A. Norris, Javier Ochoa-Repáraz, and Lloyd H. Kasper, "Credibility, Integrity, Transparency & Courage: The Haitian Cholera Outbreak and the United Nations (UN)," *Journal of Infection and Public Health* 11, no. 1 (2018): 140–141; Jocalyn Clark, "Cholera Cover Up in Haiti," *The Lancet Infectious Diseases* 17, no. 1 (2017): 38. International law has worked in the UN's favor, providing them with immunity from prosecution. See Mara Pillinger, Ian Hurd, and Michael N. Barnett, "How to Get Away with Cholera: The UN, Haiti, and International Law," *Perspectives on Politics* 14, no. 1 (2016): 70–86.

17. For example, consider how blame is apportioned in the words of a Haitian woman living in the rural border area of Ouanaminthe that we interviewed in 2017: "Cholera came and killed so many people, so many people, because there was no good water to drink."

18. See details of the situation of Haitian migrants regarding cholera in the Dominican Republic in Hunter M. Keys, Bonnie N. Kaiser, Jenny W. Foster, Matthew C. Freeman, Rob Stephenson, Andrea J. Lund, and Brandon A. Kohrt, "Cholera Control and Anti-Haitian Stigma in the Dominican Republic: From Migration Policy to Lived Experience," *Anthropology & Medicine* (2017): 1–19.

19. "Unsanitary subjects" was coined by Charles Briggs to describe those the authorities perceived as sources of disease versus "sanitary citizens" who pose no threat. See Charles L. Briggs, "Why Nation-States and Journalists Can't Teach People to Be Healthy: Power and Pragmatic Miscalculation in Public Discourses on Health," *Medical Anthropology Quarterly* 17, no. 3 (2003): 287–321.

20. The story of Kaluaiko'olau as told later by Pi'ilani, recorded in Frances N. Frazier, "True Story of Kaluaiko'olau, or Ko'olau the Leper," *The Hawaiian Journal of History* 21 (1987): 1–41.

21. Leprosy is a bacterial disease, now curable with multi-drug antibiotic therapy over a period of several months. In 2012, the number of chronic cases of leprosy was estimated at 189,000, from 5.2 million in the 1980s. Most new cases occur in India.

22. Nowadays, we know that leprosy is a bacterial infection spread through contact with nasal fluids. It is actually quite difficult to contract, spreading very slowly through the nerves, mucosa, and skin. Treatment is with antibiotics.

23. For much of written European and Middle Eastern history, leprosy was the most feared and stigmatized of all diseases. At the time, though, no one knew what caused leprous skin lesions, but divine retribution for past sins was a common explanation. People with leprosy were also confined in a huge network of specialized institutions called leprosariums, keeping the seemingly filthy, damaged, and undesirable away from the healthy, clean, and good. Stigma around leprosy decreased in the 1700s as the bacteria causing the disease was identified, treatments were developed, and education efforts publicized that it is difficult to contract. But leprosy's deep stigma had a further, energetic resurgence during the global, colonial expansions of the 1800s. As England took control of new lands, epidemics of introduced diseases such as leprosy surged in the local populations. Germ theory, new at the time, fed European ideas about the inferiority of "filthy," "uncivilized" colonized peoples who could threaten the Western world with "their" diseases. See Mary Douglas, "Witchcraft and Leprosy: Two Strategies of Exclusion," *Man* 26 (1991): 723–736.

24. Leprosy quarantine wasn't that helpful at combating the disease. Norway took the opposite approach from Hawai'i at the same time. They completely eradicated leprosy without any quarantine at all. The obvious reason why quarantine was a choice in Hawai'i but not in Norway was probably that Norwegians with leprosy were "more like" Norwegian policy makers. Ron Amundson and Akira Ruddle-Miyamoto, "A Wholesome Horror: The Stigmas of Leprosy in 19th Century Hawaii," *Disability Studies Quarterly* 30, no. 3/4 (2010).

25. Noting that Hawai'ians, at the time, bathed more often than the newer arrivals to the kingdom.

26. The former leper colony on Moloka'i is still occupied today. Within a decade or so, the last remaining patient-residents will die. Their homes will be bulldozed, and the former leprosy colony will transform into a new $40 million national park.

27. Pennie Moblo, "Institutionalising the Leper: Partisan Politics and the Evolution of Stigma in Post-Monarchy Hawai'i," *The Journal of the Polynesian Society* 107, no. 3 (1998): 229–262; R. D. K. Herman, "Out of Sight, Out of Mind, Out of Power: Leprosy, Race and Colonization in Hawai'i," *Journal of Historical Geography* 27, no. 3 (2001): 319–337.

28. This monstrous capacity to decide who will receive healthcare and who will die in any society is sometimes termed "biopower."

Chapter 4. Fat, Bad, and Everywhere

1. We use the word "fat" when describing social views of weight, and "obesity" when describing technical/clinical categories of weight.

2. For example, Jennifer Hansen, "Explode and Die! A Fat Woman's Perspective on Prenatal Care and the Fat Panic Epidemic," *Narrative Inquiry in Bioethics* 4, no. 2 (2014): 99–101. For a discussion derived from how it impacts a small sample of middle-class university students in California, see Susan Greenhalgh, "Weighty Subjects: The Biopolitics of the US War on Fat," *American Ethnologist* 39, no. 3 (2012): 471–487.

3. Marco Caliendo and Wang-Sheng Lee, "Fat Chance! Obesity and the Transition from Unemployment to Employment," *Economics & Human Biology* 11, no. 2 (2013): 121–133; Charles L. Baum and William F. Ford, "The Wage Effects of Obesity: A Longitudinal Study," *Health Economics* 13, no. 9 (2004): 885–899.

4. Obesity is technically a body mass index (BMI) of thirty or higher. Extreme (morbid) obesity is a BMI above forty.

5. Rebecca Puhl and Kelly D. Brownell, "Stigma, Discrimination, and Obesity," in *Eating Disorders and Obesity: A Comprehensive Handbook* (New York: Guilford Press, 2002), 108–112.

6. Rebecca M. Puhl and Chelsea A. Heuer, "The Stigma of Obesity: A Review and Update," *Obesity* 17, no. 5 (2009): 941–964.

7. N. A. Schvey, R. M. Puhl, K. A. Levandoski, and K. D. Brownell, "The Influence of a Defendant's Body Weight on Perceptions of Guilt," *International Journal of Obesity* 37, no. 9 (2013): 1275.

8. Christian S. Crandall, "Do Parents Discriminate against Their Heavyweight Daughters?" *Personality and Social Psychology Bulletin* 21, no. 7 (1995): 724–735.

9. Rebecca M. Puhl, Joerg Luedicke, and Cheslea Heuer, "Weight-Based Victimization Toward Overweight Adolescents: Observations and Reactions of

Peers," *Journal of School Health* 81, no. 11 (2011): 696–703; David R. Schaefer and Sandra D. Simpkins, "Using Social Network Analysis to Clarify the Role of Obesity in Selection of Adolescent Friends," *American Journal of Public Health* 104, no. 7 (2014): 1223–1229.

10. Lindsey Murtagh and David S. Ludwig, "State Intervention in Life-Threatening Childhood Obesity," *JAMA* 306, no. 2 (2011): 206–207.

11. The children's book is *Don't Call Me Fat* by Pat Thomas (2014). This was pointed out in a March 15, 2017, post by Ragen Chastain who blogs at https://danceswithfat.wordpress.com/blog/, a really excellent source for those who want to learn more about the experience of living with weight in the United States.

12. But all the advanced economies show signs of extreme stigma toward weight. For example, the Danish public are much more likely to support use of public funds to support smoking-related treatments (86 percent) than obesity-related ones (30 percent): Thomas Bøker Lund, Morten Ebbe Juul Nielsen, and Peter Sandøe, "In a Class of Their Own: The Danish Public Considers Obesity Less Deserving of Treatment Compared with Smoking-Related Diseases," *European Journal of Clinical Nutrition* 69, no. 4 (2015): 514.

13. Karin Kwambai, "Obesity Treatment: One Size Does Not Fit All," *Narrative Inquiry in Bioethics* 4, no. 2 (2014): 104–107.

14. Tara Parker-Pope, "Fat Stigma Spreads Around the Globe," last modified March 30, 2011, https://well.blogs.nytimes.com/2011/03/30/spreading-fat-stigma-around-the-globe/.

15. Kirsti Malterud and Kjersti Ulriksen, "Norwegians Fear Fatness More Than Anything Else—A Qualitative Study of Normative Newspaper Messages on Obesity and Health," *Patient Education and Counseling* 81, no. 1 (2010): 47–52.

16. "Norway PM Opens Up About Online Abuse," last modified December 1, 2015, https://www.thelocal.no/20151201/norway-pm-opens-up-about-online-abuse.

17. See the Korean data in Maddalena Marini, Natarajan Sriram, Konrad Schnabel, Norbert Maliszewski, Thierry Devos, Bo Ekehammar, Reinout Wiers, et al., "Overweight People Have Low Levels of Implicit Weight Bias, but Overweight Nations Have High Levels of Implicit Weight Bias," *PLoS One* 8, no. 12 (2013): e83543.

18. Cindi SturtzSreetharan is leading our team's efforts to understand "fat talk" around the globe, considering South Korea within a range of different countries. Engaging in the rituals of fat talk means making self-deprecating comments about your own body ("I'm fat!") that are designed to elicit supportive ("no, you're not!") interactions from friends. Fat talk has been widespread in the United States for a long time, especially by young women. Exposure to fat talk apparently triggers eating disorders, depression, and other health impacts of lowered self-esteem. However, while we know fat talk is common and normal in the United States, almost nothing has been written about whether it happens in other parts of the globe. An excellent ethnography about fat talk is in Mimi Nichter, *Fat Talk: What Girls and Their Parents Say about Dieting* (Cambridge, MA: Harvard University Press, 2001).

19. The findings are based on analysis of data for a sample of 11,492 nationally representative adults, from the Korean Nutrition and Health Examination Survey 2014 and 2009 (KNHANES). Alexandra A. Brewis, SeungYong Han, and Cindi L. SturtzSreetharan, "Weight, Gender, and Depressive Symptoms in South

Korea," *American Journal of Human Biology* 29, no. 4 (2017): e22972. SeungYong Han, Alexandra A. Brewis, and Cindi SturtzSreetharan, "Employment and Weight Status: The Extreme Case of Body Concern in South Korea," *Economics & Human Biology* 29 (2018): 115–121.

20. Alexandra A. Brewis, SeungYong Han, and Cindi L. SturtzSreetharan, "Weight, Gender, and Depressive Symptoms in South Korea," *American Journal of Human Biology* 29, no. 4 (2017): e22972.

21. The HRAF is the historic database of ethnographic work from 307 world cultures, from the Abipón to the Zuni. See http://hraf.yale.edu.

22. Peter J. Brown and Melvin Konner, "An Anthropological Perspective on Obesity," *Annals of the New York Academy of Sciences* 499, no. 1 (1987): 29–46.

23. Rebecca Popenoe, *Feeding Desire: Fatness, Beauty and Sexuality Among a Saharan People* (Abingdon, UK: Routledge, 2012).

24. Alexandra A. Brewis, Stephen T. McGarvey, J. Jones, and Boyd A. Swinburn, "Perceptions of Body Size in Pacific Islanders," *International Journal of Obesity* 22, no. 2 (1998): 185.

25. Brewis, McGarvey, Jones, and Swinburn, "Perceptions of Body Size in Pacific Islanders," 185–189.

26. Alexandra Brewis, "Biocultural Aspects of Obesity in Young Mexican Schoolchildren," *American Journal of Human Biology* 15, no. 3 (2003): 446–460.

27. Neoliberalism is based on the ideals of individualism, privatization, and decentralization. It tends to push responsibility for healthcare onto consumers and away from government, reduce oversight, and emphasize for-profit interests. In the industrialized nations, neoliberal policies are associated with the production of much greater health disparities.

28. Alexandra A. Brewis, Amber Wutich, Ashlan Falletta-Cowden, and Isa Rodriguez-Soto, "Body Norms and Fat Stigma in Global Perspective," *Current Anthropology* 52, no. 2 (2011): 269–276.

29. Sarah Krebs Council and Caitlyn Placek, "Cultural Change and Explicit Anti-Fat Attitudes in a Developing Nation: A Case Study in Rural Dominica," *Social Medicine* 9, no. 1 (2014): 11–21; Eileen P. Anderson-Fye and Alexandra Brewis, eds., *Fat Planet: Obesity, Culture, and Symbolic Body Capital* (Albuquerque: University of New Mexico Press, 2017).

30. This study is reported in Alexandra A. Brewis and Amber Wutich, "A World of Suffering? Biocultural Approaches to Fat Stigma in the Global Contexts of the Obesity Epidemic," *Annals of Anthropological Practice* 38, no. 2 (2014): 269–283.

31. Christian S. Crandall and Amy Eshleman, "A Justification-Suppression Model of the Expression and Experience of Prejudice," *Psychological Bulletin* 129, no. 3 (2003): 414.

32. Overweight is technically a BMI between 25 and 30. Obesity is technically a BMI over 30. Thus, in Paraguay, a lot of adults sit between a BMI of 25 and 30.

33. The IAT captures how much practice someone has had, cognitively, at putting two ideas together (e.g., fat + bad). If someone's ideas changed recently, the IAT might not capture that because the thought is not yet sufficiently automatic to show up as rapidly accessed. Project Implicit at Harvard has many online examples for people to self-test, including an IAT capturing anti-fat bias, at https://implicit.harvard.edu/implicit/.

34. Amy Kathleen McLennan, "An Ethnographic Investigation of Lifestyle Change, Living for the Moment, and Obesity Emergence in Nauru," PhD dissertation, University of Oxford, 2013; Jessica Hardin, Amy McLennan, and Alexandra Brewis, "Body Size, Body Norms, and Some Unintended Consequences of Obesity Intervention in the Pacific Islands," *Annals of Human Biology* 45, no 3 (2018): 285–294.

35. Jessica Hardin, "Christianity, Fat Talk, and Samoan Pastors: Rethinking the Fat-Positive-Fat-Stigma Framework," *Fat Studies* 4, no. 2 (2015): 178–196; Hardin, McLennan, Brewis, "Body Size, Body Norms," 285–94.

36. A. E. Becker, "Body Size, Social Standing, and Weight Management: The View from Fiji," in *Fat Planet: Obesity, Culture, and Symbolic Body Capital* (Albuquerque: University of New Mexico Press, 2017), 149–170.

37. Sarah Trainer, "Glocalizing Beauty: Weight and Body Image in the New Middle East," *Fat Planet* (2016).

38. Jonathan N. Maupin and Alexandra Brewis, "Food Insecurity and Body Norms Among Rural Guatemalan Schoolchildren," *American Anthropologist* 116, no. 2 (2014): 332–337.

39. Although it may seem counterintuitive, famine and food insecurity increasingly intersect with obesity. This seems to operate through many possible pathways—heightening overall stress and depression levels as people worry about their next meal, overeating in response to shortages when food is available, changes in how mothers feed their children, or encouraging pragmatic purchasing of cheaper, higher calorie foods. In many poorer sectors of the countries with rapidly growing economies, overweight and underweight are thus starting to converge as dual conditions of poverty. Moreover, the growth stunting that can result from chronic undernutrition in childhood provides a smaller frame onto which to later store excess calories, making them fatter at the same weight as someone taller. Accordingly, as many of the lower-income nations increasingly move out of poverty, food insecure generations will become increasingly placed in obesogenic environments. Tackling obesity in the global south will thus increasingly be complicated because governments are working to deliver interventions to overweight and underweight people at the same time, in the same communities, sometimes living in the very same households and even eating from the same pot. Overnutrition is usually targeted through health education, such as telling people to eat less processed food or drink. Both are most often targeted at schoolchildren. What we clearly don't need is undernourished people refusing food, or overnourished people getting unnecessary calories through feeding programs. The real challenge is that, as feeding programs directed at undernutrition began to succeed, they can roll right into encouraging unhealthy weight gain.

40. But, the children from food insecure homes, who lived with hunger, also attached some negative words to thin bodies as well.

41. In 2015, anthropologist Emily Yates-Doerr published a detailed analysis of how local people were understanding and responding to government efforts to "fight obesity" in the urban area of Xela, some three hours to the west of Acatenango. Just like in the UAE, as described by Sarah Trainer, anti-obesity action is spreading ideas about how fat is bad and unmodern. See Emily Yates-Doerr, *The Weight of Obesity: Hunger and Global Health in Postwar Guatemala* (Berkeley: University of California Press, 2015).

42. Joseph Hackman, Jonathan Maupin, and Alexandra A. Brewis, "Weight-Related Stigma Is a Significant Psychosocial Stressor in Developing Countries: Evidence from Guatemala," *Social Science & Medicine* 161 (2016): 55–60.

43. Marini, Sriram, Schnabel, Maliszewski, Devos, Ekehammar, Wiers, et al., "Overweight People Have Low Levels of Implicit Weight Bias, but Overweight Nations Have High Levels of Implicit Weight Bias," e83543. This online study of previously collected IATs from seventy-seven countries has shown that some level of anti-fat bias exists across the board based on both questionnaires and IATs (although much less in Asia). This sample is drawing only from people who are on the internet, so we would expect them to have greater exposure to mass and social media about the negative effects and meanings of weight. The results speak to a very complex cultural landscape with regard to who is explicitly and implicitly fat stigmatizing and why. Much more research is needed to sort out and properly theorize these complex trends.

Chapter 5. The Tyranny of Weight Judgment

1. This argument about the distribution of risk being shaped well outside of individual choice is detailed in chapter 4 of Alexandra A. Brewis, *Obesity: Cultural and Biocultural Perspectives* (New Brunswick: Rutgers University Press, 2010).

2. In our own work on body norms, we generally apply the idea that culture is based on consensus. That is, if most people agree with the assertion then it's a cultural fact.

3. Anja Hilbert, Winfried Rief, and Elmar Braehler, "Stigmatizing Attitudes Toward Obesity in a Representative Population-Based Sample," *Obesity* 16, no. 7 (2008): 1529–1534.

4. B. Mohammadpour-Ahranjani, M. J. Pallan, A. Rashidi, and P. Adab, "Contributors to Childhood Obesity in Iran: The Views of Parents and School Staff," *Public Health* 128, no. 1 (2014): 83–90.

5. Helen Gonçalves, David A. González, Cora P. Araújo, Ludmila Muniz, Patrícia Tavares, Maria C. Assunção, Ana MB Menezes, and Pedro C. Hallal, "Adolescents' Perception of Causes of Obesity: Unhealthy Lifestyles or Heritage?" *Journal of Adolescent Health* 51, no. 6 (2012): S46–S52.

6. Information about this study and findings can be found in Danielle M. Raves, Alexandra Brewis, Sarah Trainer, SeungYong Han, and Amber Wutich, "Bariatric Surgery Patients' Perceptions of Weight-Related Stigma in Healthcare Settings Impair Post-Surgery Dietary Adherence," *Frontiers in Psychology* 7 (2016): 1497; Alexandra Brewis, Sarah Trainer, SeungYong Han, and Amber Wutich, "Publically Misfitting: Extreme Weight and the Everyday Production and Reinforcement of Felt Stigma," *Medical Anthropology Quarterly* 31, no. 2 (2017): 257–276; Sarah Trainer, Alexandra Brewis, and Amber Wutich, "Not 'Taking the Easy Way Out': Reframing Bariatric Surgery from Low-Effort Weight Loss to Hard Work," *Anthropology & Medicine* 24, no. 1 (2017): 96–110; Sarah Trainer, Amber Wutich, and Alexandra Brewis, "Eating in the Panopticon: Surveillance of Food and Weight before and after Bariatric Surgery," *Medical Anthropology* 36, no. 5 (2017): 500–14.

7. Trainer, Wutich, and Brewis, "Eating in the Panopticon: Surveillance of Food and Weight Before and After Bariatric Surgery," 500–514.

8. Trainer, Brewis, and Wutich, "Not 'Taking the Easy Way Out': Reframing Bariatric Surgery from Low-Effort Weight Loss to Hard Work," 96–110.

9. The BMI cut points are in themselves arbitrary and/or misleading. See Daniel J. Hruschka, Craig Hadley, and Alexandra Brewis, "Disentangling Basal and Accumulated Body Mass for Cross-Population Comparisons," *American Journal of Physical Anthropology* 153, no. 4 (2014): 542–550.

10. J. L. Kraschnewski, J. Boan, J. Esposito, N. E. Sherwood, E. B. Lehman, D. K. Kephart, and C. N. Sciamanna, "Long-Term Weight Loss Maintenance in the United States," *International Journal of Obesity* 34, no. 11 (2010): 1644.

11. There are also lots of upstream and other mediating reasons why some people are more likely to gain and retain weight than others, unrelated to willpower and self-control. Genetics explain some differences in appetite and metabolism. Women are more prone to maintaining high body weights than men, everything else being equal, because their biologies are designed to grow and feed children. Where you live can influence your risk—people in neighborhoods that are safe, walkable, with access to fresh foods and parks, and excellent public transportation options tend to be slimmer. Differences in the average length of people's limbs relative to their trunk mean relative fat deposition is higher in some populations/parts of the world than others. Some medications, such as antidepressants, trigger weight gain or forestall weight loss. Newer "fetal programming" research theorizes that children who are born to underfed mothers develop fundamentally different energy metabolisms that preadapt them to live better in low food environments. If they are then exposed later to lots of calories (characterizing modern life), they are more likely to metabolize energy into fat.

12. Stanley Heshka and David B. Allison, "Is Obesity a Disease?" *International Journal of Obesity* 25, no. 10 (2001): 1401.

13. A. Janet Tomiyama, Laura E. Finch, Angela C. Incollingo Belsky, Julia Buss, Carrie Finley, Marlene B. Schwartz, and Jennifer Daubenmier, "Weight Bias in 2001 Versus 2013: Contradictory Attitudes Among Obesity Researchers and Health Professionals," *Obesity* 23, no. 1 (2015): 46–53.

14. For example, Geraldine M. Budd, Megan Mariotti, Diane Graff, and Kathleen Falkenstein, "Health Care Professionals' Attitudes About Obesity: An Integrative Review," *Applied Nursing Research* 24, no. 3 (2011): 127–137.

15. Kimberly A. Gudzune, Mary Catherine Beach, Debra L. Roter, and Lisa A. Cooper, "Physicians Build Less Rapport with Obese Patients," *Obesity* 21, no. 10 (2013): 2146–2152.

16. Michelle R. Hebl and J. Xu, "Weighing the Care: Physicians' Reactions to the Size of a Patient," *International Journal of Obesity* 25, no. 8 (2001): 1246.

17. "First Do No Harm: Real Stories of Fat Prejudice in Health Care," accessed December 28, 2017, https://fathealth.wordpress.com.

18. Lauren Moore, "I'm Your Patient, Not a Problem," *Narrative Inquiry in Bioethics* 4, no. 2 (2014): 110–112.

19. Sean M. Phelan, Diane J. Burgess, Mark W. Yeazel, Wendy L. Hellerstedt, Joan M. Griffin, and Michelle van Ryn, "Impact of Weight Bias and Stigma on Quality of Care and Outcomes for Patients with Obesity," *Obesity Reviews* 16, no. 4 (2015): 319–326. For example, Kimberly A. Gudzune, Sara N. Bleich, Thomas M. Richards, Jonathan P. Weiner, Krista Hodges, and Jeanne M. Clark, "Doctor Shopping by Overweight and Obese Patients is Associated with Increased Healthcare Utilization," *Obesity* 21, no. 7 (2013): 1328–1334.

20. Kirsti Malterud and Kjersti Ulriksen, "Obesity, Stigma, and Responsibility in Health Care: A Synthesis of Qualitative Studies," *International Journal of Qualitative Studies on Health and Well-being* 6, no. 4 (2011): 8404.

21. Daniel S. Goldberg, "Fatness, Medicalization, and Stigma: On the Need to do Better," *Narrative Inquiry in Bioethics* 4, no. 2 (2014): 117–123.

22. Alexandra A. Brewis, "Stigma and the Perpetuation of Obesity," *Social Science & Medicine* 118 (2014): 152–158.

23. Sarah Trainer, Alexandra Brewis, Deborah Williams, and Jose Rosales Chavez, "Obese, Fat, or 'Just Big?' Young Adult Deployment of and Reactions to Weight Terms," *Human Organization* 74, no. 3 (2015): 266–275.

24. Meg Bruening, Punam Ohri-Vachaspati, Alexandra Brewis, Melissa Laska, Michael Todd, Daniel Hruschka, David R. Schaefer, Corrie M. Whisner, and Genevieve Dunton, "Longitudinal Social Networks Impacts on Weight and Weight-Related Behaviors Assessed Using Mobile-Based Ecological Momentary Assessments: Study Protocols for the SPARC Study," *BMC Public Health* 16, no. 1 (2016): 901; Alexandra Brewis, Stephanie Brennhofer, Irene van Woerden, and Meg Bruening, "Weight Stigma and Eating Behaviors on a College Campus: Are Students Immune to Stigma's effects?" *Preventive Medicine Reports* 4 (2016): 578–584.

25. Some findings are reported in Alexandra A. Brewis and Amber Wutich, "A World of Suffering? Biocultural Approaches to Fat Stigma in the Global Contexts of the Obesity Epidemic," *Annals of Anthropological Practice* 38, no. 2 (2014): 269–283; Alexandra Brewis, Stephanie Brennhofer, Irene van Woerden, and Meg Bruening, "Weight Stigma and Eating Behaviors on a College Campus: Are Students Immune to Stigma's Effects?" *Preventive Medicine Reports* 4 (2016): 578–584.

26. We suspect that weight stigma on other less diverse, more elite campuses would be much higher than at ASU.

27. Natasha A. Schvey, Rebecca M. Puhl, and Kelly D. Brownell, "The Impact of Weight Stigma on Caloric Consumption," *Obesity* 19, no. 10 (2011): 1957–1962; Also see Brenda Major, Jeffrey M. Hunger, Debra P. Bunyan, and Carol T. Miller, "The Ironic Effects of Weight Stigma," *Journal of Experimental Social Psychology* 51 (2014): 74–80.

28. We did not find the same for eating, we think because undergraduate freshman eating patterns are so completely disordered anyway. Brewis, Brennhofer, Woerden, and Bruening, "Weight Stigma," 578–584.

29. For example, Dianne Neumark-Sztainer, Melanie Wall, Mary Story, and Amber R. Standish, "Dieting and Unhealthy Weight Control Behaviors During Adolescence: Associations with 10-Year Changes in Body Mass Index," *Journal of Adolescent Health* 50, no. 1 (2012): 80–86.

30. Angela C. Incollingo Rodriguez, Courtney M. Heldreth, and A. Janet Tomiyama, "Putting on Weight Stigma: A Randomized Study of the Effects of Wearing a Fat Suit on Eating, Well-Being, and Cortisol," *Obesity* 24, no. 9 (2016): 1892–1898.

31. For example, a large study of Australian adults showed that those who felt more stressed gained more weight in a five-year period, taking into account lifestyle factors such as diet and exercise. Jessica L. Harding, Kathryn Backholer, Emily D. Williams, Anna Peeters, Adrian J. Cameron, Matthew J. L. Hare,

Jonathan E. Shaw, and Dianna J. Magliano, "Psychosocial Stress is Positively Associated with Body Mass Index Gain over 5 Years: Evidence from the Longitudinal AusDiab Study," *Obesity* 22, no. 1 (2014): 277–286.

32. Jason D. Seacat, Sarah C. Dougal, and Dooti Roy, "A Daily Diary Assessment of Female Weight Stigmatization," *Journal of Health Psychology* 21, no. 2 (2016): 228–240.

33. Seacat, Dougal, Roy, "A Daily Diary," 228–240.

34. We have explained how this works in detail elsewhere: Brewis, "Stigma and the Perpetuation," 152–158.

35. Rebecca M. Puhl and Kelly D. Brownell, "Confronting and Coping with Weight Stigma: An Investigation of Overweight and Obese Adults," *Obesity* 14, no. 10 (2006): 1802–1815.

36. Natalie Boero, "All the News That's Fat to Print: The American 'Obesity Epidemic' and the Media," *Qualitative Sociology* 30, no. 1 (2007): 41–60.

37. George Parker, "Mothers at Large: Responsibilizing the Pregnant Self for the 'Obesity Epidemic,'" *Fat Studies* 3, no. 2 (2014): 101–118.

38. Shona Hilton, Chris Patterson, and Alison Teyhan, "Escalating Coverage of Obesity in UK Newspapers: The Evolution and Framing of the 'Obesity Epidemic' from 1996 to 2010," *Obesity* 20, no. 8 (2012): 1688–1695.

39. Sei-Hill Him and L. Anne Willis, "Talking About Obesity: News Framing of Who is Responsible for Causing and Fixing the Problem," *Journal of Health Communication* 12, no. 4 (2007): 359–376.

40. Amy Luke and Richard S. Cooper, "Physical Activity Does Not Influence Obesity Risk: Time to Clarify the Public Health Message," *International Journal of Epidemiology* 42, no. 6 (2013): 1831–1836.

41. Abigail C. Saguy, *What's Wrong with Fat?* (Oxford, UK: Oxford University Press, 2012).

42. Vivianne Clark, "New Government will have to Act on Obesity, Donal O'Shea Says," *Irish Times*, April 1, 2016, http://www.irishtimes.com/news/health/new -government-will-have-to-act-on-obesity-donal-o-shea-says-1.2595039.

43. Independent.ie, "Ireland's Obesity Problem will be Worse than Cholera or AIDS for our Health Service, Professor Warns," last modified May 6, 2015, http://www.independent.ie/irish-news/health/irelands-obesity-problem-will-be -worse-than-cholera-or-aids-for-our-health-service-professor-warns-31199764 .html.

44. J. Maher, "Shifting the Weight Around: The 'Childhood Obesity Epidemic and Maternal Responsibility,'" *The Australian Sociological Association (TASA)* (2008): 1–17.

45. L. Rokas, "Meet 15-Year-Old Ballerina Lizzy Who Challenges Body Stereotypes in Dance," accessed November 11, 2017, http://www.boredpanda .com/challenging-body-stereotypes-ballerina-lizzy/.

46. Emma Gray, "Proof That You Can Be a Wildly Talented Dancer at Any Size," *Huffington Post*, February 5, 2014, http://www.huffingtonpost.com/2014/02 /05/fat-girl-dancing-video-talk-dirty-to-me_n_4730408.html.

47. "These Overweight Dancers Prove Everyone Wrong," Star2.com, November 30, 2016, http://www.star2.com/culture/arts/2016/11/30/cuba -overweight-dancers/.

48. Emma Rich, "'I See Her Being Obesed!': Public Pedagogy, Reality Media and the Obesity Crisis," *Health* 15, no. 1 (2011): 3–21.

49. Sarah E. Domoff, Nova G. Hinman, Afton M. Koball, Amy Storfer-Isser, Victoria L. Carhart, Kyoung D. Baik, and Robert A. Carels, "The Effects of Reality Television on Weight Bias: An Examination of The Biggest Loser," *Obesity* 20, no. 5 (2012): 993–998.

50. Domoff, Hinman, Koball, Storfer-Isser, Carhart, Baik, Carels, "The Effects of Reality," 993–998; Samantha Thomas, Jim Hyde, and Paul Komesaroff, "'Cheapening the Struggle': Obese People's Attitudes towards the Biggest Loser," *Obesity Management* 3, no. 5 (2007): 210–215.

51. Jina H. Yoo, "No Clear Winner: Effects of The Biggest Loser on the Stigmatization of Obese Persons," *Health Communication* 28, no. 3 (2013): 294–303.

52. Gina Kolata, "After 'The Biggest Loser,' Their Bodies Fought to Regain Weight," *New York Times*, May 2, 2016, https://www.nytimes.com/2016/05/02/health/biggest-loser-weight-loss.html; Meredith Jacobs, "'Biggest Loser' Contestants Given Drugs to Lose Weight? NBC Reportedly Looks into Allegations," *Newsweek*, July 19, 2018, https://www.newsweek.com/biggest-loser-nbc-investigation-drug-use-dr-robert-huizenga-defamation-1031756.

53. Sarah Trainer, Alexandra Brewis, Amber Wutich, Liza Kurtz, and Monet Niesluchowski, "The Fat Self in Virtual Communities: Success and Failure in Weight-Loss Blogging," *Current Anthropology* 57, no. 4 (2016): 523–528.

54. Kim D. Raine, Candace I. J. Nykiforuk, Karen Vu-Nguyen, Laura M. Nieuwendyk, Eric VanSpronsen, Shandy Reed, and T. Cameron Wild, "Understanding Key Influencers' Attitudes and Beliefs about Healthy Public Policy Change for Obesity Prevention," *Obesity* 22, no. 11 (2014): 2426–2433.

55. Aneel Karnani, Brent McFerran, and Anirban Mukhopadhyay, "Corporate Leanwashing and Consumer Beliefs About Obesity," *Current Nutrition Reports* 6, no. 3 (2017): 206–211; Daniel G. Aaron and Michael B. Siegel, "Sponsorship of National Health Organizations by Two Major Soda Companies," *American Journal of Preventive Medicine* 52, no. 1 (2017): 20–30.

56. Gabriele Ciciurkaite and Brea L. Perry, "Body Weight, Perceived Weight Stigma and Mental Health Among Women at the Intersection of Race/Ethnicity and Socioeconomic Status: Insights from the Modified Labelling Approach," *Sociology of Health & Illness* 40, no. 1 (2018): 18–37.

Chapter 6. World War O

1. We have had many extended discussions on this point over the last few years with Lt General Benjamin Freakley (ret.). He spent part of his long military career as Master of Infantry at Fort Benning. He explained that, not only does obesity limit recruiting into the military, but also a major fitness problem for active soldiers because they often gain significant weight while deployed. See Mission: Readiness—Military Leaders for Kids, *Too Fat to Fight* (Washington, DC: Mission: Readiness, 2010), http://cdn.missionreadiness.org/MR_Too_Fat_to_Fight-1.pdf; John Cawley and Johanna Catherine Maclean, "Unfit for Service: The Implications of Rising Obesity for US Military Recruitment," *Health Economics* 21, no. 11 (2012): 1348–1366. Popkin discusses how it is also a security issue in China and Mexico. See Barry M. Popkin, "Is the Obesity Epidemic a National Security

Issue around the Globe?" *Current Opinion in Endocrinology, Diabetes, and Obesity* 18, no. 5 (2011): 328–331.

2. Jeffrey M. Friedman, "A War on Obesity, Not the Obese," *Science* 299, no. 5608 (2003): 856–858.

3. Marie Ng, Tom Fleming, Margaret Robinson, Blake Thomson, Nicholas Graetz, Christopher Margono, and Erin C. Mullany, "Global, Regional, and National Prevalence of Overweight and Obesity in Children and Adults During 1980–2013: A Systematic Analysis for the Global Burden of Disease Study 2013," *The Lancet* 384, no. 9945 (2014): 766–781.

4. Some Pacific Islands (like Nauru) have no data made available and might otherwise have been on this list. These "fattest countries" lists are really a form of national shaming. So, it is no surprise they are disinterested in sharing the relevant statistics with the World Health Organization.

5. Jack Woodfield, "Introducing Images of Rotten Teeth on Fizzy Drinks Could Encourage Healthier Choices," accessed May 27, 2018, https://www.diabetes.co.uk /news/2018/may/introducing-images-of-rotten-teeth-on-fizzy-drinks-could -encourage-healthier-choices-92712561.html.

6. The 2004 World Health Organization *Global Strategy on Diet, Physical Activity and Health* recommends that individuals achieve energy balance and a healthy weight, limit total fats and shift consumption from saturated to unsaturated, try to eliminate trans-fatty acids, eat more fruits, vegetables, legumes, whole grains, and nuts, drink less sugar and limit salt, have at least thirty minutes of regular, moderate-intensity physical activity on most days. Some countries coming closer to the guidelines in national policy are Georgia, Mongolia, and the Republic of Moldova. Carl Lachat, Stephen Otchere, Dominique Roberfroid, Abubakari Abdulai, Florencia Maria Aguirre Seret, Jelena Milesevic, Godfrey Xuereb, Vanessa Candeias, and Patrick Kolsteren, "Diet and Physical Activity for the Prevention of Noncommunicable Diseases in Low- and Middle-Income Countries: A Systematic Policy Review," *PLoS Medicine* 10, no. 6 (2013): e1001465.

7. Maria Suurballe, "LazyTown Teaches Kids to Pick Fruit Over Chocolate," accessed May 10, 2018, http://www.playthegame.org/upload/magazine2007/pdf /pages/playthegamemagazine07pg27.pdf.

8. "Fit for Purpose," *The Economist*, March 29, 2007, http://www.economist .com/node/8922395.

9. "Obesity Update 2017," OECD.org, accessed May 10, 2018, http://www .oecd.org/els/health-systems/Obesity-Update-2017.pdf.

10. For examples of LiveLighter's "toxic fat" campaign see "About Toxic Fat," accessed May 10, 2018, https://livelighter.com.au/The-Facts/About-Toxic-Fat.

11. Lizzie Parry, "'Put Pictures of Fat People on Junk Food to Show the Dangers': Experts Say Rising Obesity Levels Pose Greater Heath Risk Than Smoking," *Daily Mail*, May 19, 2014, http://www.dailymail.co.uk/health/article -2632675/The-food-industry-regulated-like-tobacco-Experts-say-rising-obesity -levels-poses-greater-health-risk-smoking.html.

12. Lindsay F. Wiley, "Shame, Blame, and the Emerging Law of Obesity Control," *UC Davis Law Review* 47 (2013): 121–188.

13. J. Variyam, "Nutrition Labeling in the Food-Away-From-Home Sector. An Economic Assessment," USDA Research Report 4 (2015). There is a recent

trend toward insurance discounts or other incentives for those employees who exhibit the "right" health behaviors and reaching toward such measures as lower weight. Apparently, 90 percent of companies using this approach used weight as one of the main targets. This is legal in the United States because weight is considered by the government as modifiable by individuals.

14. World Health Organization, *Global Strategy on Diet, Physical Activity and Health*, accessed March 1, 2019, http://www.who.int/dietphysicalactivity/childhood _why/en/.

15. George Parker, "Mothers at Large: Responsibilizing the Pregnant Self for the 'Obesity Epidemic,'" *Fat Studies* 3, no. 2 (2014): 101–118.

16. For example, David J. P. Barker, Keith M. Godfrey, Peter D. Gluckman, Jane E. Harding, Julie A. Owens, and Jeffrey S. Robinson, "Fetal Nutrition and Cardiovascular Disease in Adult Life," *The Lancet* 341, no. 8850 (1993): 938–941.

17. A. Wiggins, "Professor calls for end to fertility treatment weight limit," *New Zealand Herald*, July 26, 2017. For some similar concerns around Australian policies see Newsdesk, "End 'unjust' fertility treatment ban for obese women: report," Flinders University, March 17, 2017, https://news.flinders.edu.au/blog /2017/03/17/end-unjust-fertility-treatment-ban-for-obese-women-report/.

18. Emma Amanda Harper and Geneviève Rail, "'Gaining the Right Amount for my Baby': Young Pregnant Women's Discursive Constructions of Health," *Health Sociology Review* 21, no. 1 (2012): 69–81.

19. Darren Powell and Katie Fitzpatrick, "'Getting Fit Basically Just Means, like, Nonfat': Children's Lessons in Fitness and Fatness," *Sport, Education and Society* 20, no. 4 (2015): 463–484.

20. Dooley, Jennifer Allyson Dooley, Sameer Deshpande, and Carol E. Adair, "Comparing Adolescent-Focused Obesity Prevention and Reduction Messages," *Journal of Business Research* 63, no. 2 (2010): 154–160.

21. Melissa Healy, "Small Steps, Ad Council and U.S. Department of Health & Human Services," *LA Times*, January 2, 2006, http://www.latimes.com/health/la-he -behavior2jan02-story.html.

22. Rebecca Puhl, Joerg Luedicke, and Jamie Lee Peterson, "Public Reactions to Obesity-Related Health Campaigns: A Randomized Controlled Trial," *American Journal of Preventive Medicine* 45, no. 1 (2013): 36–48; Courtney C. Simpson, "Investigating the Effects of Obesity Prevention Campaigns," master's thesis, Virginia Commonwealth University, 2015, http://scholarscompass.vcu.edu/etd/3702.

23. Gary M. Lucas Jr, "Paternalism and Psychic Taxes: The Government's Use of Negative Emotions to Save Us from Ourselves," *S. Cal. Interdisc. LJ* 22 (2012): 227.

24. Sarah Trainer, Alexandra Brewis, Deborah Williams, and Jose Rosales Chavez, "Obese, Fat, or 'Just Big'? Young Adult Deployment of and Reactions to Weight Terms," *Human Organization* 74, no. 3 (2015): 266–275.

25. Joe Piggin and Jessica Lee, "'Don't Mention Obesity': Contradictions and Tensions in the UK Change4Life Health Promotion Campaign," *Journal of Health Psychology* 16, no. 8 (2011): 1151–1164.

26. Rebecca Puhl, Jamie Lee Peterson, and Joerg Luedicke, "Fighting Obesity or Obese Persons? Public Perceptions of Obesity-Related Health Messages," *International Journal of Obesity* 37, no. 6 (2013): 774.

27. Paul Campos, "Michelle Obama's Let's Move Campaign is Helping Bullies," *The Daily Beast* 16 (2011).

28. Emma Rich and John Evans, "'Fat Ethics'—The Obesity Discourse and Body Politics," *Social Theory & Health* 3, no. 4 (2005): 341–358.

29. Jan Wright and Valerie Harwood, eds., *Biopolitics and the 'Obesity Epidemic': Governing Bodies*, vol. 3 (Abingdon, UK: Routledge, 2012).

30. For example, Kristen Cooksey-Stowers, Marlene B. Schwartz, and Kelly D. Brownell, "Food Swamps Predict Obesity Rates Better than Food Deserts in the United States," *International Journal of Environmental Research and Public Health* 14, no. 11 (2017): 1366.

31. Roland Sturm and Aiko Hattori, "Diet and obesity in Los Angeles County 2007–2012: Is there a measurable effect of the 2008 'Fast-Food Ban'?" *Social Science & Medicine* 133 (2015): 205–211.

32. Food deserts are areas which people have insufficient access to fresh, healthy, affordable food.

33. Alexandra Brewis and Meredith Gartin, "Biocultural Construction of Obesogenic Ecologies of Childhood: Parent-Feeding versus Child-Eating Strategies," *American Journal of Human Biology* 18, no. 2 (2006): 203–213.

34. It may even be a sensible health trade-off, since so many studies show that feeling connected, supported, accepted, and understood are as important to health as is good nutrition.

35. Moreover, these strategies don't work very well: In 2011, the government of Denmark introduced a tax on foods such as cheese, butter, and pizza. By 2012, the tax had been repealed, following taxpayer protest—and the observed reality—that Danes continued purchasing high fat foods, but from across the border in Germany where the costs were lower. See Ned Stafford, "Denmark Cancels 'Fat Tax' and Shelves 'Sugar Tax' Because of Threat of Job Losses," *BMJ: British Medical Journal (Online)* 345 (2012).

36. Ketevan Rtveladze, Tim Marsh, Simon Barquera, Luz Maria Sanchez Romero, David Levy, Guillermo Melendez, Laura Webber, Fanny Kilpi, Klim McPherson, and Martin Brown, "Obesity Prevalence in Mexico: Impact on Health and Economic Burden," *Public Health Nutrition* 17, no. 1 (2014): 233–239.

37. This is a hot-button political issue in part because these rates skyrocketed under president Vicente Fox, formerly the CEO of Coca-Cola in Mexico. During his time running the company, sales in Mexico increased by almost 50 percent.

38. ANSA was heavily shaped by the World Health Organization's *Global Strategy on Diet, Physical Activity and Health.*

39. In order, flavored milk beverages, sugar-sweetened soda, high-fat milk, agua fresca (fruit water), and sugared coffee/tea.

40. "Obesity Update," OECD.org.

41. Lauren Villagran, "Lucha Libre: A Spandex-Clad Campaign Against Obesity in Mexico," *Christian Science Monitor*, September 4, 2012, http://www.csmonitor.com /World/Americas/2012/0904/Lucha-Libre-A-spandex-clad-campaign-against -obesity-in-Mexico.

42. The World Health Organization has been very active in promoting directly to governments the need to curtail the powerful role of Big Food, Big Drink, and Big Snack in making us fat. The corporations that are often the target of these

efforts (such as Coca-Cola or Kraft) spend huge amounts on advertising and marketing in developing nations. And such companies recognize that poorer sectors of lower-income countries can be targeted through marketing as a huge and growing market for low-margin, high-volume, highly processed foods, with potentially massive profits. This focus on "blaming the multinational" is an attractive pitch to legislators. Limiting junk food advertising on television comes at no cost to the government. Requiring menu warnings and food packaging labels passes the cost and effort directly to the companies. Taxing consumer purchases of junk food and sweetened drinks generates additional revenue. Anything that nudges behavior change is going to be easier—and cheaper—than direct and focused interventions with individuals. Yet, on the other hand, the science suggests these legislative efforts often fail to yield any real and meaningful results in improving health. Moreover, it seems such approaches also have encouraged industry-funded research that is more likely to suggest other approaches may be more effective, as a means to derail efforts that place responsibility on Big Food. For a detailed discussion, see Marion Nestle, *Unsavory Truth: How Food Companies Skew the Science of What We Eat* (New York: Basic Books, 2018).

43. M. Arantxa Colchero, Juan Rivera-Dommarco, Barry M. Popkin, and Shu Wen Ng, "In Mexico, Evidence of Sustained Consumer Response Two Years After Implementing a Sugar-Sweetened Beverage Tax," *Health Affairs* 36, no. 3 (2017): 564–571; M. Arantxa Colchero, Barry M. Popkin, Juan A. Rivera, and Shu Wen Ng, "Beverage Purchases from Stores in Mexico Under the Excise Tax on Sugar Sweetened Beverages: Observational Study," *BMJ* 352 (2016): h6704. Other economic analyses suggest little or no change, for example, Simón Barquera, Ismael Campos, and Juan A. Rivera, "Mexico Attempts to Tackle Obesity: The Process, Results, Push Backs and Future Challenges," *Obesity Reviews* 14 (2013): 69–78. Economists suggest such "sin taxes" just further decrease spending power among the poorest, who spend a much larger percentage of income on food, since they tend to keep purchasing the less healthy foods regardless. See Benjamin B. Lockwood, and Dmitry Taubinsky, *Regressive Sin Taxes*, no. w23085 (National Bureau of Economic Research, 2017); Mark Fox, Tracey Anderson, Sue Anderson, and April Black, "Food Taxes: Can You Control Behavior and Health Outcomes through Taxation?" *American Journal of Medical Research* 4, no. 1 (2017): 93. Moreover, small taxes, such as applied in Mexico don't seem to work well for "fat taxing." Only large taxes seem to actually result in changes in obesity risk at the population level. See Caroline Franck, Sonia M. Grandi, and Mark J. Eisenberg, "Taxing Junk Food to Counter Obesity," *American Journal of Public Health* 103, no. 11 (2013): 1949–1953.

44. Andreia Azevedo Soares, "Putting Taxes into the Diet Equation," *Bulletin of the World Health Organization* 94, no. 4 (2016): 239.

45. Jaime Tomás Page Pliego, "Refresco y Diabetes Entre los Mayas de Tenejapa, San Cristóbal de Las Casas y Chamula, Chiapas," *LiminaR* 11, no. 1 (2013): 118–133.

46. Alexandra Brewis and Sarah Lee, "Children's Work, Earnings, and Nutrition in Urban Mexican Shantytowns," *American Journal of Human Biology* 22, no. 1 (2010): 60–68. Our study included extended focal follows of extremely low-income informal community children in the time spent outside home and

school with focus on foraging and working for cash, and assessments of children's diet and food sharing. It was conducted in the late 1990s.

47. Similarly, we found that children working for cash spent nearly 100 percent of their cash income on junk food. The decision to buy fried snacks and cookies wasn't so much about hunger (as even the poorest households could produce tortillas to fill a stomach), as about the ability of sharing to solidify friendships. See Sarah Lee and Alexandra Brewis, "Children's Autonomous Food Acquisition in Mexican Shantytowns," *Ecology of Food and Nutrition* 48, no. 6 (2009): 435–456.

48. In the 1970s, the Coca-Cola Company was successful in shifting Chiapas rituals that historically focused on rum to use Coke instead. See June Nash, "Consuming Interests: Water, Rum, and Coca-Cola from Ritual Propitiation to Corporate Expropriation in Highland Chiapas," *Cultural Anthropology* 22, no. 4 (2007): 621–639.

49. Alex Myers, David Fig, Aviva Tugendhaft, Jessie Mandle, Jonathan Myers, and Karen Hofman, "Sugar and Health in South Africa: Potential Challenges to Leveraging Policy Change," *Global Public Health* 12, no. 1 (2017): 98–115.

50. The cases like Samoa and Paraguay show us that just confusing the "fat is bad" message could help. We need more research directly testing if introducing and supporting counter-models related to "fat is good" that create greater ambiguity around the meanings of big bodies sufficient to reduce felt stigma. This might work because it at least gives people options for how they are allowed to present themselves and relate to others. Supporting the international scope and scale of fat acceptance activism but intersecting it with local traditions that embrace positive attributes of large bodies, would be another approach worth testing.

51. Emily Mendenhall, H. Stowe McMurry, Roopa Shivashankar, KM Venkat Narayan, Nikhil Tandon, and Dorairaj Prabhakaran, "Normalizing Diabetes in Delhi: A Qualitative Study of Health and Health Care," *Anthropology & Medicine* 23, no. 3 (2016): 295–310.

52. In a large, randomized, controlled cluster trial in Germany, providing water fountains with refillable bottles in school reduced consumption of caloric drinks and some overweight risk. Rebecca Muckelbauer, Lars Libuda, Kerstin Clausen, André Michael Toschke, Thomas Reinehr, and Mathilde Kersting, "Promotion and Provision of Drinking Water in Schools for Overweight Prevention: Randomized, Controlled Cluster Trial," *Pediatrics* 123, no. 4 (2009): e661–e667.

Chapter 7. Once Crazy, Always Crazy

1. Sokratis Dinos, Scott Stevens, Marc Serfaty, Scott Weich, and Michael King, "Stigma: The Feelings and Experiences of 46 People with Mental Illness: Qualitative Study," *The British Journal of Psychiatry* 184, no. 2 (2004): 176–181.

2. Hearing they have a schizophrenic mother or brother, family members can also find themselves pitied or shamed because of the idea they need to "carry" the "useless" person for decades. Or discover they, too, are stigmatized, because of the idea that mental illness runs in families.

3. Alex J. Mitchell, Davy Vancampfort, Amber De Herdt, Weiping Yu, and Marc De Hert, "Is the Prevalence of Metabolic Syndrome and Metabolic

Abnormalities Increased in Early Schizophrenia? A Comparative Meta-Analysis of First Episode, Untreated and Treated Patients," *Schizophrenia Bulletin* 39, no. 2 (2012): 295–305.

4. Sing Lee, Marcus Y. L. Chiu, Adley Tsang, Helena Chui, and Arthur Kleinman, "Stigmatizing Experience and Structural Discrimination Associated with the Treatment of Schizophrenia in Hong Kong," *Social Science & Medicine* 62, no. 7 (2006): 1685–1696.

5. Elaine Brohan, Rodney Elgie, Norman Sartorius, Graham Thornicroft, and GAMIAN-Europe Study Group, "Self-Stigma, Empowerment and Perceived Discrimination among People with Schizophrenia in 14 European Countries: The GAMIAN-Europe Study," *Schizophrenia Research* 122, no. 1–3 (2010): 232–238.

6. Anthropologist Sue Estroff spent eighteen months in the mid-1970s doing fieldwork with forty-three people being treated for schizophrenia and other severe mental illnesses in Madison, Wisconsin. They were part of this new wave of patients, managed through a program called the Program of Assertive Community Treatment (PACT). The focus was on teaching people how to create "normal" daily lives: working, caring for themselves, socializing, and integrating into their families. Estroff spent time in the outpatient clinic and the program's social and sport activities but also visited their homes, ate with them, went camping or played pool with them, and tracked them down on the streets. She hung out, too, with the program staff. For six weeks, she took the same treatment that many of her respondents were taking, a drug called fluphenazine. But the side effects made normal interaction with others who didn't understand the signs difficult—like the leg jiggling, facial grimacing, and eye rolling. The result was that the treated patients, too, became labeled as "crazy" regardless. Sue E. Estroff, *Making It Crazy: An Ethnography of Psychiatric Clients in an American Community* (Berkeley: University of California Press, 1985). These side effects are seen much more frequently with older antipsychotics, currently more often used in developing countries. New drugs cause fewer side effects.

7. Gro Harlem Brundtland, "Mental Health: New Understanding, New Hope," *Jama* 286, no. 19 (2001): 2391.

8. Diana Rose, Graham Thornicroft, Vanessa Pinfold, and Aliya Kassam, "250 Labels Used to Stigmatise People with Mental Illness," *BMC Health Services Research* 7, no. 1 (2007): 97.

9. Time to Change, "I can Stand my Mental Illnesses at Work, but not the Discrimination," accessed April 8, 2017, http://www.time-to-change.org.uk/blog/i -can-stand-my-mental-illnesses-work-not-discrimination.

10. Erving Goffman, *Asylums: Essays on the Social Situation of Mental Patients and Other Inmates* (New York: Anchor Books, 1961).

11. Estimates range between 5'1" and 5'6" as his adult height.

12. Goffman published *"The Presentation of Self in Everyday Life"* in 1957 based on his PhD dissertation.

13. Goffman, *Asylums*, 1961. Goffman's *Asylums* got real attention and spurred some change around abuses in mental health treatment. Even so, stigma was slow to change in mental health treatment circles.

14. Especially Thomas S. Szasz, "The Myth of Mental Illness," *American Psychologist* 15, no. 2 (1960): 113.

15. Destigmatization first began to emerge as a stated goal in mental illness treatment in the late 1950s. Particularly after the UK Percy Report of 1957 concluded that mental disorders should be regarded "in much the same way physical illness or disability"—a theme that has shaped much of what came after. But it took a while for destigmatization to be recognized as necessary for mental illness *treatment*. For much of Western European history, mental illnesses like schizophrenia were viewed as a moral problem. Lines between criminality and "madness" were blurry. The causes of prostitution, blasphemy, and insanity were thought to be borne of sin, character weakness, and other individual failings. Equating illness with moral and spiritual failure is a core part of the stigma process. Early asylums, as places to put away those who were seen as crazy, were infamously abusive. Bethlehem Royal Hospital, a psychiatric hospital founded in London during the medieval era is the best known case. Treatments included beatings, restraint in chains, and isolation. In time, Bedlam, a local nickname for the hospital, became synonymous with lunacy, squalor, and chaos. The emergence of a new, more medicalized view of mental illness as a "brain disease" from the mid-1800s removed some of this stigma that led to people being hidden away in places like Bedlam. But it also encouraged other new stigmas. By becoming understood as a "disease like any other", it also promoted the idea that mental illness was an incurable mental condition. Punishment and restraint in "mad-houses" morphed into medical treatment in hospitals. But it didn't mean the abuse stopped. When some people have power over other people with few rights, mistreatment often happens. In psychiatric hospitals, abuses included the use of unnecessary and cruel treatments like chemical or physical restraints, and the widespread use of electroconvulsive therapy (ECT) and lobotomy right up until the 1970s. Inhumane mental illness treatment continued to fulfill an important social function, just as dreadful lunatic asylums had in prior centuries. Everyone knew: if you didn't follow the social rules, you'd be taken away.

16. Erving Goffman, *Stigma: Notes on the Management of Spoiled Identity* (New York: Simon and Schuster, 2009).

17. Based on archival materials (http://cdclv.unlv.edu/ega/), it seems that Goffman did later change some of his ideas, particularly after he spent several years caring for a mentally ill, suicidal wife. Although he never admitted to any connection with his personal life, he began to acknowledge that maybe mental illness was sometimes a medical problem in need of a medical treatment. But his ideas about the importance of labeling—and that mental illness is learned through the rituals and norms of treatment—remain highly influential.

18. Fiscal realities also made community-based treatment attractive as social policy. So, in the late 1970s–1980s, there was a rapid shift to moving treatment for mental illness out of the hospital. Community reintegration has often also created new stigma as it turned out, of the not-in-my-backyard variety.

19. For example, Jim Van Os, "'Salience Syndrome' Replaces 'Schizophrenia' in DSM-V and ICD-11: Psychiatry's Evidence-Based Entry Into the 21st Century?" *Acta Psychiatrica Scandinavica* 120, no. 5 (2009): 363–372.

20. Patrick W. Corrigan, "Erasing Stigma Is Much More Than Changing Words," *Psychiatric Services* 65, no. 10 (2014): 1263–1264.

21. At least according to a study of attitudes of 259 university students in Shinsuke Koike, Sosei Yamaguchi, Yasutaka Ojio, Takafumi Shimada, Kei-ichiro

Watanabe, and Shuntaro Ando, "Long-Term Effect of a Name Change for Schizophrenia on Reducing Stigma," *Social Psychiatry and Psychiatric Epidemiology* 50, no. 10 (2015): 1519–1526; Sosei Yamaguchi, Masashi Mizuno, Yasutaka Ojio, Utako Sawada, Asami Matsunaga, Shuntaro Ando, and Shinsuke Koike, "Associations Between Renaming Schizophrenia and Stigma-Related Outcomes: A Systematic Review," *Psychiatry and Clinical Neurosciences* 71, no. 6 (2017): 347–362.

22. Ai Aoki, Yuta Aoki, Robert Goulden, Kiyoto Kasai, Graham Thornicroft, and Claire Henderson, "Change in Newspaper Coverage of Schizophrenia in Japan Over 20-Year Period," *Schizophrenia Research* 175, no. 1–3 (2016): 193–197.

23. Steve Silberman, *Neurotribes: The Legacy of Autism and the Future of Neurodiversity* (New York: Penguin, 2015).

24. Laurent Mottron, "Changing Perceptions: The Power of Autism," *Nature* 479, no. 7371 (2011): 33.

25. Peter S. Jensen, David Mrazek, Penelope K. Knapp, Laurence Steinberg, Cynthia Pfeffer, John Schowalter, and Theodore Shapiro, "Evolution and Revolution in Child Psychiatry: ADHD as a Disorder of Adaptation," *Journal of the American Academy of Child & Adolescent Psychiatry* 36, no. 12 (1997): 1672–1681.

26. Thomas Armstrong, "The Myth of the Normal Brain: Embracing Neurodiversity," *AMA Journal of Ethics* 17, no. 4 (2015): 348–352.

27. Michael Bernick, "Increasing Autism Employment: An Anthropologist's Perspective," accessed May, 9, 2017, https://www.forbes.com/sites/michaelbernick/2017/05/09/the-anthropologist-of-autism-employment/#76bea2756153.

28. Bruce G. Link, Francis T. Cullen, Elmer Struening, Patrick E. Shrout, and Bruce P. Dohrenwend, "A Modified Labeling Theory Approach to Mental Disorders: An Empirical Assessment," *American Sociological Review* (1989): 400–423.

29. For example, Sigrun Olafsdottir and Bernice A. Pescosolido, "Constructing Illness: How the Public in Eight Western Nations Respond to a Clinical Description of 'Schizophrenia,'" *Social Science & Medicine* 73, no. 6 (2011): 929–938.

30. Jo C. Phelan, Bruce G. Link, Ann Stueve, and Bernice A. Pescosolido, "Public Conceptions of Mental Illness in 1950 and 1996: What Is Mental Illness and Is It to Be Feared?" *Journal of Health and Social Behavior* (2000): 188–207.

31. Matthias C. Angermeyer and Herbert Matschinger, "Causal Beliefs and Attitudes to People with Schizophrenia: Trend Analysis Based on Data from Two Population Surveys in Germany," *The British Journal of Psychiatry* 186, no. 4 (2005): 331–334.

32. And, because biogenetic explanations emphasize the idea that mental illness tends to run in families, it can also result in greater—rather than lesser—courtesy stigma (that is, stigma by association) attaching to the family. Erlend P. Kvaale, Nick Haslam, and William H. Gottdiener, "The 'Side Effects' of Medicalization: A Meta-Analytic Review of How Biogenetic Explanations Affect Stigma," *Clinical Psychology Review* 33, no. 6 (2013): 782–794.

33. A review of a wide range of studies suggests that reeducation works best with adolescents. Perhaps this is because their ideas about mental illness are less entrenched than that of adults', and so they are more likely to accept new ways of viewing it. Patrick W. Corrigan, Scott B. Morris, Patrick J. Michaels, Jennifer D. Rafacz, and Nicolas Rüsch, "Challenging the Public Stigma of Mental Illness: A Meta-Analysis of Outcome Studies," *Psychiatric Services* 63, no. 10 (2012): 963–973.

A major issue is that the effects of educational campaigns are normally only measured in weeks or months. Long-term impacts are hard to demonstrate. But it seems, without constant reinforcement or other support, they wear off quickly.

34. Elaine Cumming and John Cumming, *Closed Ranks: An Experiment in Mental Health Education* (Cambridge, MA: Harvard University Press, 1957).

35. Alan Rosen, Garry Walter, Dermot Casey, and Barbara Hocking, "Combating Psychiatric Stigma: An Overview of Contemporary Initiatives," *Australasian Psychiatry* 8, no. 1 (2000): 19–26.

36. P. K. Maulik, S. Devarapalli, S. Kallakuri, A. Tewari, S. Chilappagari, M. Koschorke, and G. Thornicroft, "Evaluation of an Anti-Stigma Campaign Related to Common Mental Disorders in Rural India: A Mixed Methods Approach," *Psychological Medicine* (2016): 1–11.

37. Beate Schulze, "Stigma and Mental Health Professionals: A Review of the Evidence on an Intricate Relationship," *International Review of Psychiatry* 19, no. 2 (2007): 137–155.

38. Bettina Friedrich, Sara Evans-Lacko, Jillian London, Danielle Rhydderch, Claire Henderson, and Graham Thornicroft, "Anti-Stigma Training for Medical Students: The Education Not Discrimination Project," *The British Journal of Psychiatry* 202, no. s55 (2013): s89–s94.

39. Of course, it is more complex than just pushing psychiatrists to be more empathetic, or even changing how they diagnose and treat patients. Psychiatrists themselves are stigmatized, too. Over the decades, film has often cast the psychiatrist as madman himself. They are almost invariably portrayed negatively—such as neurotic, uncaring, self-absorbed, addicted, or rigid men. Friends and family worry they are themselves being analyzed or assume the work is dreadful and avoid asking questions. Their own medical colleagues suggest that are in a "soft medicine," suitable for those who shrink from the sight of blood. Therapy is seen as "something anyone can do" compared to the intricacies of surgery. And they know their important work is undervalued and under resourced simply because of the patients treated by their specialty. They watch their heart surgeon friends get the best hospital facilities and more research funding and better tests paid for by insurance and know exactly why.

40. Corrigan, Morris, Michaels, Rafacz, and Rüsch, "Challenging the Public Stigma of Mental Illness."

41. Jane Eddy, Lynette A. Hart, and Ronald P. Boltz, "The Effects of Service Dogs on Social Acknowledgments of People in Wheelchairs," *The Journal of Psychology* 122, no. 1 (1988): 39–45.

42. And empathy-building strategies seem best for full adults; they are typically a bust with adolescents—for all the reasons any parent of a normal teen might understand. Corrigan, Morris, Michaels, Rafacz, and Rüsch, "Challenging the Public Stigma of Mental Illness."

43. Sing Lee, Margaret TY Lee, Marcus YL Chiu, and Arthur Kleinman, "Experience of Social Stigma by People with Schizophrenia in Hong Kong," *The British Journal of Psychiatry* 186, no. 2 (2005): 153–157.

44. At different times and places, mental health services have considered that placing people with mental disorders in the community should help them. It didn't. One study of two halfway houses in Germany showed residents were unable

to connect with their neighbors and ended up living in a de facto "complementary ghetto" after their neighbors rejected them. Matthias C. Angermeyer, Bruce G. Link, and Alice Majcher-Angermeyer, "Stigma Perceived by Patients Attending Modern Treatment Settings: Some Unanticipated Effects of Community Psychiatry Reforms," *Journal of Nervous and Mental Disease* 175, no. 1 (1987): 4–11.

45. Shuntaro Ando, Sarah Clement, Elizabeth Alexandra Barley, and Graham Thornicroft, "The Simulation of Hallucinations to Reduce the Stigma of Schizophrenia: A Systematic Review," *Schizophrenia Research* 133, no. 1–3 (2011): 8–16.

46. Brooke Shields, "War of Words," *New York Times*, July 1, 2005, http://www .nytimes.com/2005/07/01/opinion/war-of-words.html.

47. Bipolar disorder, like unipolar depression, is marked by periods of low mood with a high degree of subjective distress. But these fluctuate with episodes of elevated, irritable, expansive manic mood. Something like 1–5 percent of people will have the condition in their lifetime, and onset is usually in the early twenties.

48. Wendy Cross and Ken Walsh, "Star Shots: Stigma, Self Disclosure and Celebrity in Bipolar Disorder," in *Bipolar Disorder—A Portrait of a Complex Mood Disorder*, ed. J. Barnhill (Rijeka, Croatia: In Tech, 2012), 221–236.

49. Peter Cram, A. Mark Fendrick, John Inadomi, Mark E. Cowen, Daniel Carpenter, and Sandeep Vijan, "The Impact of a Celebrity Promotional Campaign on the Use of Colon Cancer Screening: The Katie Couric Effect," *Archives of Internal Medicine* 163, no. 13 (2003): 1601–1605.

50. Corrigan, Morris, Michaels, Rafacz, and Rüsch, "Challenging the Public Stigma of Mental Illness." An interesting case in the age of social media was a #ShoutYourAbortion Twitter campaign of 2015. Although intended to destigmatize abortion, over a quarter of the 7,639 responding tweets to those who linked the hashtag were subject to stigma. Moral reactions included allusions to sin, outright disgust, and calls for them to bleed to death. Kami Kosenko, Emily Winderman, and Abigail Pugh, "The Hijacked Hashtag: The Constitutive Features of Abortion Stigma in the #ShoutYourAbortion Twitter Campaign," *International Journal of Communication* 13 (2019): 1–21.

51. Randall M. Packard, Ruth L. Berkelman, Howard Frumkin, and Peter J. Brown, eds., *Emerging Illnesses and Society: Negotiating the Public Health Agenda* (Baltimore: Johns Hopkins University Press, 2004).

52. B. Hocking, "StigmaWatch: Tackling Stigma Against Mental Illness and Suicide in The Media: a SANE Report," *SANE: Australia* (2013). Cited in H. Stuart, "Reducing the Stigma of Mental Illness," *Global Mental Health* 3 (2016).

53. Joe Wright, "Only Your Calamity: The Beginnings of Activism by and for People with AIDS," *American Journal of Public Health* 103, no. 10 (2013): 1788–1798.

54. Josh Gamson, "Silence, Death, and the Invisible Enemy: AIDS Activism and Social Movement 'Newness,'" *Social Problems* 36, no. 4 (1989): 351–367.

55. Anish P. Mahajan, Jennifer N. Sayles, Vishal A. Patel, Robert H. Remien, Daniel Ortiz, Greg Szekeres, and Thomas J. Coates, "Stigma in the HIV/AIDS Epidemic: A Review of the Literature and Recommendations for the Way Forward," *AIDS (London, England)* 22, suppl 2 (2008): S67.

56. Deborah B. Gould, "ACT UP, Racism, and the Question of How to Use History," *Quarterly Journal of Speech* 98, no. 1 (2012): 54–62.

57. This idea of disease and their stigma "settling into" poor or marginalized communities is from Paul Farmer, *Infections and Inequalities: The Modern Plagues* (Berkeley: University of California Press, 2001).

58. Stuart, "Reducing the Stigma of Mental Illness."

59. Nadia Kadri and Norman Sartorius, "The Global Fight Against the Stigma of Schizophrenia," *PLoS Medicine* 2, no. 7 (2005): e136.

60. Heather Stuart, "Fighting the Stigma Caused by Mental Disorders: Past Perspectives, Present Activities, and Future Directions," *World Psychiatry* 7, no. 3 (2008): 185–188.

61. Open the Doors, "Stories from Canada," accessed April 9, 2017, http://openthedoors.com/english/04_04.html.

62. Starting in 1997, New Zealand's "Like Minds, Like Mine" campaign has tried to do better, learning from OTD's failures. Yet, in 2011, one thousand users of mental health services were asked about their experiences of mental health stigma in the prior five years. Nearly all respondents reported feeling stigma in some way within the last year, such as being shunned (26 percent) or keeping their hidden their condition because they anticipated discrimination (57 percent). The worst stigma was from families. The main improvement they reported as a result of the campaign was better treatment when they were accessing government services like unemployment. But, while half of those using mental health services surveyed thought things had got better in the previous five years, the other half thought stigma was much the same or worse. The more recent English "Time to Change" (TTC) campaign, launched in 2008, took the need for measurable outcomes seriously. It aimed for "a 5 percent positive shift in public attitudes towards mental health problems and a 5 percent reduction in discrimination" with "100 000 people with mental health problems to have increased knowledge, confidence and assertiveness" by 2012. Spending over £21 million in three years, it mainly focused on social marketing, such as tv advertisements. The website uses personal stories, provides advice on the need to step in and help "your mates" if they are acting differently, and asks people to pledge their commitment to challenging stigma. The key messages included "mental illnesses are common," "people with them can lead meaningful lives," "that the stigma can be worse than the illness itself" and "we can all do something to help people with mental illness." Based on the idea that social contact matters, they trained people wearing "Time to Change" t-shirts to strike up conversations with spectators at sporting events, in supermarket checkout lines, or to start threads online at fanzines or other social pages. Yet, based on better tracking of outcomes, the results of TTC are also equivocal at best. People using mental health services reported small reductions in experiences of discrimination. Medical students showed a positive, but short-lived, change in attitudes. Worse, surveys conducted at the start and end of the campaign suggested that public opinions did not change for the better. And those with mental illness said clinicians didn't treat them any better either. Press coverage of positive stories about people with mental illness increased. But at the same time, negative stories also continued to appear. Press coverage in Great Britain simply became more polarized. Calum Thornicroft, Allan Wyllie, Graham Thornicroft, and Nisha Mehta, "Impact of the 'Like Minds, Like Mine' Anti-Stigma and Discrimination Campaign in New

Zealand on Anticipated and Experienced Discrimination," *Australian & New Zealand Journal of Psychiatry* 48, no. 4 (2014): 360–370; Claire Henderson, Sara Evans-Lacko, and Graham Thornicroft, "Mental Illness Stigma, Help Seeking, and Public Health Programs," *American Journal of Public Health* 103, no. 5 (2013): 777–780; Lee Knifton and Neil Quinn, "Media, Mental Health and Discrimination: A Frame of Reference for Understanding Reporting Trends," *International Journal of Mental Health Promotion* 10, no. 1 (2008): 23–31; Time to Change, "Time to Change. Let's End Mental Health Discrimination," accessed April 9, 2017, http://www.time-to-change.org.uk; SeeMeScotland, "See Me So Far. A Review of the First 4 Years of the Scottish Anti-Stigma Campaign," accessed April 9, 2017, http://www.docs.csg.ed.ac.uk/EqualityDiversity/see_me_so_far.pdf.

63. Corrigan, Morris, Michaels, Rafacz, and Rüsch, "Challenging the Public Stigma of Mental Illness." More recently, the larger anti-stigma efforts are focusing in on the idea that telling positive *stories* is the key. These should highlight the idea that people with mental illness are competent, reliable, contribute, and have meaningful lives. They are heroes for dealing with the adversity that mental illness brings. For example, the two-week Scottish Mental Health Arts and Film Festival highlights music, film, comedy, literature, and theater by people with mental illness. This approach, which brings the public into contact with those affected, seems to have had some measured success. Some of the offerings seem to decrease stigmatizing fear immediately after. But at least one film increased it. N. Quinn, A. Shulman, L. Knifton, and P. Byrne, "The Impact of a National Mental Health Arts and Film Festival on Stigma and Recovery," *Acta Psychiatrica Scandinavica* 123, no. 1 (2011): 71–81. And the long-term—positive and negative—impacts of these types of community-outreach events aren't apparent, because no one is tracking them.

64. Graham Thornicroft, Nisha Mehta, Sarah Clement, Sara Evans-Lacko, Mary Doherty, Diana Rose, Mirja Koschorke, Rahul Shidhaye, Claire O'Reilly, and Claire Henderson, "Evidence for Effective Interventions to Reduce Mental-Health-Related Stigma and Discrimination," *The Lancet* 387, no. 10023 (2016): 1123–1132.

65. For example, Dianne E. Green, Iain A. McCormick, Frank H. Walkey, and Antony JW Taylor, "Community Attitudes to Mental Illness in New Zealand Twenty-Two Years On," *Social Science & Medicine* 24, no. 5 (1987): 417–422.

66. Kathleen M. Griffiths, Bradley Carron-Arthur, Alison Parsons, and Russell Reid, "Effectiveness of Programs for Reducing the Stigma Associated with Mental Disorders. A Meta-Analysis of Randomized Controlled Trials," *World Psychiatry* 13, no. 2 (2014): 161–175.

67. Brundtland, "Mental Health," 2391.

68. Norman Sartorius, "One of the Last Obstacles to Better Mental Health Care: The Stigma of Mental Illness," in *The Image of Madness* (Basel, Switzerland: Karger Publishers, 1999): 96–104.

69. Graham Thornicroft, Nisha Mehta, Sarah Clement, Sara Evans-Lacko, Mary Doherty, Diana Rose, Mirja Koschorke, Rahul Shidhaye, Claire O'Reilly, and Claire Henderson, "Evidence for Effective Interventions to Reduce Mental-Health-Related Stigma and Discrimination," *The Lancet* 387, no. 10023 (2016): 1123–1132.

70. Brandon A. Kohrt and Ian Harper, "Navigating Diagnoses: Understanding Mind–Body Relations, Mental Health, and Stigma in Nepal," *Culture, Medicine, and*

Psychiatry 32, no. 4 (2008): 462; Gerald T. Keusch, Joan Wilentz, and Arthur Kleinman, "Stigma and Global Health: Developing a Research Agenda," *The Lancet* 367, no. 9509 (2006): 525–527.

Chapter 8. The Myth of the Destigmatized Society

1. Alex Cohen, Vikram Patel, R. Thara, and Oye Gureje, "Questioning an Axiom: Better Prognosis for Schizophrenia in the Developing World?" *Schizophrenia Bulletin* 34, no. 2 (2007): 229–244.

2. Details of the study are provided in Kim Hopper, Glynn Harrison, Aleksandar Janca, and Norman Sartorius, eds., *Recovery from Schizophrenia: An International Perspective: A Report from the WHO Collaborative Project, the International Study of Schizophrenia* (Oxford: Oxford University Press, 2007).

3. Conclusion, in Hopper, Harrison, Janca, Sartorius, *Recovery from Schizophrenia*.

4. Assen Jablensky and Norman Sartorius, "What Did the WHO Studies Really Find?" *Schizophrenia Bulletin* 34, no. 2 (2008): 253–255.

5. Benedetto Saraceno and Shekhar Saxena, "Mental Health Resources in the World: Results from Project Atlas of the WHO," *World Psychiatry* 1, no. 1 (2002): 40.

6. Kim Hopper and Joseph Wanderling, "Revisiting the Developed Versus Developing Country Distinction in Course and Outcome in Schizophrenia: Results from ISoS, the WHO Collaborative Followup Project," *Schizophrenia Bulletin* 26, no. 4 (2000): 835–846.

7. Antonio Lasalvia, Elena Penta, Norman Sartorius, and Scott Henderson, "Should the Label 'Schizophrenia' be Abandoned?" *Schizophrenia Research* 162, no. 1–3 (2015): 276–284.

8. Kazuo Ogawa, Mahito Miya, Akio Wataral, Masao Nakazawa, Shuichi Yuasa, and Hiroshi Utena, "A Long-Term Follow-Up Study of Schizophrenia in Japan—With Special Reference to the Course of Social Adjustment," *The British Journal of Psychiatry* 151, no. 6 (1987): 758–765; P. W. H. Lee, F. Lieh-Mak, K. K. Yu, and J. A. Spinks, "Patterns of Outcome in Schizophrenia in Hong Kong," *Acta Psychiatrica Scandinavica* 84, no. 4 (1991): 346–352; W. F. Tsoi and K. E. Wong, "A 15-year Follow-Up Study of Chinese Schizophrenic Patients," *Acta Psychiatrica Scandinavica* 84, no. 3 (1991): 217–220.

9. Nancy E. Waxler, "Is Outcome for Schizophrenia Better in Nonindustrial Societies? The Case of Sri Lanka," *Journal of Nervous and Mental Disease* 167, no. 3 (1979): 144–158. Notably, Waxler didn't explicitly use the term "stigma."

10. Michaeline Bresnahan, Paulo Menezes, Vijoy Varma, and Ezra Susser, "Geographical Variation in Incidence, Course and Outcome of Schizophrenia: A Comparison of Developing and Developed Countries," in *The Epidemiology of Schizophrenia* (Cambridge: Cambridge University Press, 2002), 18–33; Neely Laurenzo Myers, "Culture, Stress and Recovery from Schizophrenia: Lessons from the Field for Global Mental Health," *Culture, Medicine, and Psychiatry* 34, no. 3 (2010): 500–528.

11. This implication is outlined critically by Bernice A. Pescosolido, Jack K. Martin, J. Scott Long, Sigrun Olafsdottir, Karen Kafadar, and Tait R. Medina, "The Theory of Industrial Society and Cultural Schemata: Does the 'Cultural Myth of Stigma' Underlie the WHO Schizophrenia Paradox?" *American Journal of Sociology* 121, no. 3 (2015): 783–825.

12. Robert B. Edgerton and Alex Cohen, "Culture and Schizophrenia: The DOSMD Challenge," *The British Journal of Psychiatry* 164, no. 2 (1994): 222–231.

13. Roger O. A. Makanjuola and Sunday A. Adedapo, "The DSM-III Concepts of Schizophrenic Disorder and Schizophreniform Disorder a Clinical and Prognostic Evaluation," *The British Journal of Psychiatry* 151, no. 5 (1987): 611–618.

14. Jane M. Murphy, "Psychiatric Labeling in Cross-Cultural Perspective," *Science* 191, no. 4231 (1976): 1019–1028.

15. Karen Lynne Schmidt, *A Biocultural Perspective on Schizophrenic Communication in New Zealand and Papua New Guinea* (Berkeley: University of California, 1997); Karen L. Schmidt, Felix Y. Attah Johnson, and John S. Allen, "Cross-Cultural Analysis of Eventfulness in the Lives of People with Schizophrenia," *Schizophrenia Bulletin* 26, no. 4 (2000): 825–834.

16. There are some cultural differences in how the symptoms exactly manifest. The auditory hallucinations of schizophrenia are more likely to manifest for Americans as (harsh) voices, while they are kinder or playful in Ghana and India and more likely to belong to kin. Tanya M. Luhrmann, Ramachandran Padmavati, Hema Tharoor, and Akwasi Osei, "Differences in Voice-Hearing Experiences of People with Psychosis in the USA, India and Ghana: Interview-Based Study," *The British Journal of Psychiatry* 206, no. 1 (2015): 41–44.

17. Bernice A. Pescosolido, Tait R. Medina, Jack K. Martin, and J. Scott Long, "The 'Backbone' of Stigma: Identifying the Global Core of Public Prejudice Associated with Mental Illness," *American Journal of Public Health* 103, no. 5 (2013): 853–860.

18. Kaaren Mathias, Michelle Kermode, Miguel San Sebastian, Mirja Koschorke, and Isabel Goicolea, "Under the Banyan Tree—Exclusion and Inclusion of People with Mental Disorders in Rural North India," *BMC Public Health* 15, no. 1 (2015): 446. This same story is told in *Vita*, João Biehl's emotionally grueling ethnography of the life of a single "mad" woman in the favelas of Brazil. João Biehl, *Vita: Life in a Zone of Social Abandonment* (Berkeley: University of California Press, 2013). And it's clear in Jinhua Guo's recent ethnography *Stigma*, about people receiving mental health treatment in China. Jinhua Guo, *Stigma: An Ethnography of Mental Illness and HIV/AIDS in China* (Singapore: World Scientific, 2016).

19. Mathias, Kermode, Sebastian, Koschorke, Goicolea, "Under the Banyan Tree," 446.

20. Maosheng Ran, Mengze Xiang, Mingsheng Huang, and Youhe Shan, "Natural Course of Schizophrenia: 2-Year Follow-Up Study in a Rural Chinese Community," *The British Journal of Psychiatry* 178, no. 2 (2001): 154–158.

21. John S. Allen, "Are Traditional Societies Schizophrenogenic?" *Schizophrenia Bulletin* 23, no. 3 (1997): 357–364. One proposition is that a shaman's roles in traditional societies, which include seeing between this world and others, provide such a possible niche. But a detailed analysis of what a shaman actually does shows it is a complex role unsuitable for most severely mentally ill people. Lyle B. Steadman and Craig T. Palmer, "Visiting Dead Ancestors: Shamans as Interpreters of Religious Traditions," *Zygon* 29, no. 2 (1994): 173–189.

22. Roger J. Sullivan, John S. Allen, Karen L. Nero, Robert Barrett, Robert Harland, Francis X. Hezel, Marina Myles-Worsley, et al., "Schizophrenia in Palau: A Biocultural Analysis," *Current Anthropology* 48, no. 2 (2007): 189–213.

23. Roger Sullivan suggests that the very particular and intense reciprocal social interactions of clan-based life on Palau require high levels of social competence and sophistication. It is also a close-knit, smaller-scale society in which people are tied to each other through a complex set of social and economic obligations. For example, at first birthday parties, clans try to outdo each other in terms of generosity of gifts. Lower clans even sometimes take out mortgages to put on weddings and other events that match those of high clans.

24. Helena Hansen, Philippe Bourgois, and Ernest Drucker, "Pathologizing Poverty: New Forms of Diagnosis, Disability, and Structural Stigma Under Welfare Reform," *Social Science & Medicine* 103 (2014): 76–83.

25. Eileen P. Anderson-Fye and Alexandra Brewis, eds., *Fat Planet: Obesity, Culture, and Symbolic Body Capital* (Albuquerque: University of New Mexico Press, 2017).

26. Nadia Kadri and Norman Sartorius, "The Global Fight against the Stigma of Schizophrenia," *PLoS Medicine* 2, no. 7 (2005): e136.

Chapter 9. Completely Depressing

1. Ashley Hagaman, "A Critical Investigation of Suicide Surveillance Data: Exploring the Institutional and Cultural Shaping of Death in Nepal" (PhD diss., Arizona State University, 2016).

2. World Health Organization, *Suicide Rates Data by Country* (Geneva: World Health Organization, 2015).

3. The specific signs of depression show some local variation, too. In Haiti, where we are currently collecting data on women's responses to legal injustice, "thinking too much" is a local idiom that signals their distress and depression. Hagaman used a locally adapted version of the PHQ-9. Brandon A. Kohrt, Nagendra P. Luitel, Prakash Acharya, and Mark J. D. Jordans, "Detection of Depression in Low Resource Settings: Validation of the Patient Health Questionnaire (PHQ-9) and Cultural Concepts of Distress in Nepal," *BMC Psychiatry* 16, no. 1 (2016): 58.

4. Perhaps 50 percent of those diagnosed with an anxiety disorder also meet the criteria for depression. Physical symptoms can include terrifying heart palpitations, sweating, dizziness, shortness of breath, and a sense that you are dying. N. M. Batelaan, F. Smit, R. De Graaf, A. J. L. M. Van Balkom, W. A. M. Vollebergh, and A. T. F. Beekman, "Identifying Target Groups for the Prevention of Anxiety Disorders in the General Population," *Acta Psychiatrica Scandinavica* 122, no. 1 (2010): 56–65.

5. World Health Organization, *Global Health Estimates 2015: Disease Burden by Cause, Age, Sex, by Country and by Region, 2000–2015* (Geneva: World Health Organization, 2016).

6. World Health Organization, *Mental Health Services in Liberia: Building Back Better* (Geneva: World Health Organization, 2016); Sharon Alane Abramowitz, *Searching for Normal in the Wake of the Liberian War* (Philadelphia: University of Pennsylvania Press, 2014).

7. Dickens Akena, Seggane Musisi, John Joska, and Dan J. Stein, "The Association between Aids Related Stigma and Major Depressive Disorder among HIV-Positive Individuals in Uganda," *PLoS One* 7, no. 11 (2012): e48671.

8. William W. Dressler, Kathryn S. Oths, and Clarence C. Gravlee, "Race and Ethnicity in Public Health Research: Models to Explain Health Disparities," *Annual Review of Anthropology* 34 (2005): 231–252; Clarence C. Gravlee, "How Race Becomes Biology: Embodiment of Social Inequality," *American Journal of Physical Anthropology* 139, no. 1 (2009): 47–57.

9. Sunita Dodani and Rukhsana Wamiq Zuberi, "Center-Based Prevalence of Anxiety and Depression in Women of the Northern Areas of Pakistan," *Journal of Pakistan Medical Association* 50, no. 5 (2000): 138–140.

10. Craig Hadley, Alexandra Brewis, and Ivy Pike, "Does Less Autonomy Erode Women's Health? Yes. No. Maybe," *American Journal of Human Biology* 22, no. 1 (2010): 103–110.

11. Lesley Jo Weaver and Sarah Trainer, "Shame, Blame, and Status Incongruity: Health and Stigma in Rural Brazil and the Urban United Arab Emirates," *Culture, Medicine, and Psychiatry* 41, no. 3 (2017): 319–340.

12. Kathryn S. Oths, Adriana Carolo, and José Ernesto Dos Santos, "Social Status and Food Preference in Southern Brazil," *Ecology of Food and Nutrition* 42, no. 4–5 (2003): 303–324; Alexander Edmonds, *Pretty Modern: Beauty, Sex, and Plastic Surgery in Brazil* (Durham, NC: Duke University Press, 2010).

13. Lesley Jo Weaver and Craig Hadley, "Moving Beyond Hunger and Nutrition: A Systematic Review of the Evidence Linking Food Insecurity and Mental Health in Developing Countries," *Ecology of Food and Nutrition* 48, no. 4 (2009): 263–284.

14. Jonathan Stieglitz, Eric Schniter, Christopher von Rueden, Hillard Kaplan, and Michael Gurven, "Functional Disability and Social Conflict Increase Risk of Depression in Older Adulthood Among Bolivian Forager-Farmers," *Journals of Gerontology Series B: Psychological Sciences and Social Sciences* 70, no. 6 (2014): 948–956.

15. Bonnie N. Kaiser, Emily E. Haroz, Brandon A. Kohrt, Paul A. Bolton, Judith K. Bass, and Devon E. Hinton, "'Thinking Too Much': A Systematic Review of a Common Idiom of Distress," *Social Science & Medicine* 147 (2015): 170–183.

16. Jonathan Stieglitz, Adrian V. Jaeggi, Aaron D. Blackwell, Benjamin C. Trumble, Michael Gurven, and Hillard Kaplan, "Work to Live and Live to Work: Productivity, Transfers, and Psychological Well-Being in Adulthood and Old Age," in *Sociality, Hierarchy, Health: Comparative Biodemography: A Collection of Papers* (Washington, DC: National Academies Press, 2014), 197–221.

17. Lawrence H. Yang, Fang-pei Chen, Kathleen Janel Sia, Jonathan Lam, Katherine Lam, Hong Ngo, Sing Lee, Arthur Kleinman, and Byron Good, "'What Matters Most': A Cultural Mechanism Moderating Structural Vulnerability and Moral Experience of Mental Illness Stigma," *Social Science & Medicine* 103 (2014): 84–93.

18. Awareness is key. People with intellectual disabilities are one of the most overtly stigmatized groups. They have to deal everyday with bullying, extreme social rejection, and even hate crimes. But people living with intellectual disabilities vary in their awareness of what is going on. Some are fully aware and others much less so. This can be due to higher versus lower functioning. And, because intellectual disabilities are often fully under the wing of others, family and friends may openly share with them their condition—or deny it and keep

them fully in the dark. English people with intellectual disabilities were interviewed about their awareness of their impairment. And they were asked if they felt "people talk down to me," "people on the street make fun of me," and "people treat me like a child." It turns out that those who were less aware of their intellectual disabilities were much less likely to be despondent about their future and had higher self-esteem. And they had many more signs of depression and anxiety. Afia Ali, Michael King, Andre Strydom, and Angela Hassiotis, "Self-Reported Stigma and Symptoms of Anxiety and Depression in People with Intellectual Disabilities: Findings from a Cross Sectional Study in England," *Journal of Affective Disorders* 187 (2015): 224–231.

19. The notion of "unsanitary subjects" is from Briggs's work on cholera in Venezuela discussed in chapter 3. See Charles L. Briggs, *Stories in the Time of Cholera: Racial Profiling During a Medical Nightmare* (Berkeley: University of California Press, 2003).

20. Bob Bolin, Sara Grineski, and Timothy Collins, "The Geography of Despair: Environmental Racism and the Making of South Phoenix, Arizona, USA," *Human Ecology Review* 12, no. 2 (2005): 156–168.

21. Danya E. Keene, and Mark B. Padilla, "Race, Class and the Stigma of Place: Moving to 'Opportunity' in Eastern Iowa," *Health & Place* 16, no. 6 (2010): 1216–1223.

22. Amber Wutich, Alissa Ruth, Alexandra Brewis, and Christopher Boone, "Stigmatized Neighborhoods, Social Bonding, and Health," *Medical Anthropology Quarterly* 28, no. 4 (2014): 556–577. In 2013, when we did the study, anti-immigrant sentiment was riding high in Arizona. When we first began working in South Phoenix in 2006, it felt to us like a place on the rise—Arizona was booming as a construction economy and there was lots of work. Migrants and their families were arriving (mostly from Mexico) to what felt like a welcoming, booming city. But by 2010, when we started doing a new set of house-to-house surveys for a project on migrant families, we felt the sudden chill. The recession had by then settled in, the housing boom was done, and blue-collar construction jobs were gone with it. But it was the passage of SB1070, the Support Our Law Enforcement and Safe Neighborhoods Act, that hurt the most. This new law made it a misdemeanor crime for anyone to be in Arizona without carrying the required visa documents. Suddenly police could check legal status of anyone during any "lawful stop, detention or arrest." South Phoenix, with its large migrant population, seemed to be particularly targeted. Many families packed up and left for other states they saw as more welcoming. Foreclosures were rife. Families who couldn't move, hunkered down.

23. World Population Review, "Scottsdale, Arizona Population 2018," http://worldpopulationreview.com/us-cities/scottsdale-population/.

24. Average depressive symptom score based on the Brief Symptom Inventory (BSI) scale of 7.88 (±8.1) for South Phoenix versus 5.42 (±5.4) for other Latinx-predominate neighborhoods, significant at $p<0.01$. Amber Wutich, Alissa Ruth, Alexandra Brewis, and Christopher Boone, "Stigmatized Neighborhoods, Social Bonding, and Health," *Medical Anthropology Quarterly* 28, no. 4 (2014): 556–577.

25. But see Loïc J. D. Wacquant, "Urban Outcasts: Stigma and Division in the Black American Ghetto and the French Urban Periphery," *International Journal of Urban and Regional Research* 17, no. 3 (1993): 366–383; Loïc Wacquant, "Territorial

Stigmatization in the Age of Advanced Marginality," *Thesis Eleven* 91, no. 1 (2007): 66–77; Loïc Wacquant, Tom Slater, and Virgílio Borges Pereira, "Territorial Stigmatization in Action," *Environment and Planning A* 46, no. 6 (2014): 1270–1280; João Queirós and Virgílio Borges Pereira, "Voices in the Revolution: Resisting Territorial Stigma and Social Relegation in Porto's Historic Centre (1974–1976)," *The Sociological Review* 66, no. 4 (2018): 857–876; Danya E. Keene, Amy B. Smoyer, and Kim M. Blankenship, "Stigma, Housing and Identity after Prison," *The Sociological Review* 66, no. 4 (2018): 799–815.

26. Zachary Steel, Claire Marnane, Changiz Iranpour, Tien Chey, John W. Jackson, Vikram Patel, and Derrick Silove, "The Global Prevalence of Common Mental Disorders: A Systematic Review and Meta-Analysis 1980–2013," *International Journal of Epidemiology* 43, no. 2 (2014): 476–493. Women had higher period and lifetime prevalence rates for mood and anxiety disorders compared with men. Men had higher pooled prevalence rates for substance disorders than women.

27. Women are more likely to face extreme poverty because of more unpaid work, fewer assets, violence, discrimination, less educational opportunity, and all the other factors that prevent them having equal access to decently paid work. Globally, women earn almost half that of men.

28. The case of Egyptian women's trials with infertility and their desperate quests to have children is detailed in Marcia Inhorn's ethnography. Marcia C. Inhorn, *Infertility and Patriarchy: The Cultural Politics of Gender and Family Life in Egypt* (Philadelphia: University of Pennsylvania Press, 1996); Marcia C. Inhorn, *Quest for Conception: Gender, Infertility, and Egyptian Medical Traditions* (Philadelphia: University of Pennsylvania Press, 1994).

29. Sabina Faiz Rashid and Stephanie Michaud, "Female Adolescents and Their Sexuality: Notions of Honour, Shame, Purity and Pollution During the Floods," *Disasters* 24, no. 1 (2000): 54–70.

30. Mary C. Ellsberg, "Violence against Women: A Global Public Health Crisis," *Scandinavian Journal of Public Health* 34, no. 1 (2006): 1–4.

31. Liying Zhang, Xiaoming Li, Bo Wang, Zhiyong Shen, Yuejiao Zhou, Jinping Xu, Zhenzhu Tang, and Bonita Stanton, "Violence, Stigma and Mental Health among Female Sex Workers in China: A Structural Equation Modeling," *Women & Health* 57, no. 6 (2017): 685–704; Yan Hong, Chen Zhang, Xiaoming Li, Wei Liu, and Yuejiao Zhou, "Partner Violence and Psychosocial Distress among Female Sex Workers in China," *PloS One* 8, no. 4 (2013): e62290.

32. Claudia García-Moreno, Henrica AFM Jansen, Mary Ellsberg, Lori Heise, and Charlotte Watts, *WHO Multi-Country Study on Women's Health and Domestic Violence Against Women: Initial Results on Prevalence, Health Outcomes and Women's Responses* (Geneva: World Health Organization, 2005).

33. Any form of bullying or victimization can have long-term negative effects on mental health. See Andre Sourander, John Ronning, Anat Brunstein-Klomek, David Gyllenberg, Kirsti Kumpulainen, Solja Niemelä, and Hans Helenius, "Childhood Bullying Behavior and Later Psychiatric Hospital and Psychopharmacologic Treatment: Findings from the Finnish 1981 Birth Cohort Study," *Archives of General Psychiatry* 66, no. 9 (2009): 1005–1012.

34. Peilian Chi, Xiaoming Li, Junfeng Zhao, and Guoxiang Zhao, "Vicious Circle of Perceived Stigma, Enacted Stigma and Depressive Symptoms among

Children Affected by HIV/AIDS in China," *AIDS and Behavior* 18, no. 6 (2014): 1054–1062.

35. IPS Correspondents, "HIV/AIDS-CHINA: Henan Orphans Finally Speak Out," http://www.ipsnews.net/2005/03/hiv-aids-china-henan-orphans-finally-speak-out/; Guoxiang Zhao, Xiaoming Li, Xiaoyi Fang, Junfeng Zhao, Hongmei Yang, and Bonita Stanton, "Care Arrangements, Grief and Psychological Problems Among Children Orphaned by AIDS in China," *AIDS Care* 19, no. 9 (2007): 1075–1082.

36. Qun Zhao, Xiaoming Li, Linda M. Kaljee, Xiaoyi Fang, Bonita Stanton, and Liying Zhang, "AIDS Orphanages in China: Reality and Challenges," *AIDS Patient Care and STDs* 23, no. 4 (2009): 297–303; Zhonghu He and Chengye Ji, "Nutritional Status, Psychological Well-Being and the Quality of Life of AIDS Orphans in Rural Henan Province, China," *Tropical Medicine & International Health* 12, no. 10 (2007): 1180–1190.

37. Kimberle Crenshaw, "Demarginalizing the Intersection of Race and Sex: A Black Feminist Critique of Antidiscrimination Doctrine, Feminist Theory and Antiracist Politics," *University of Chicago Legal Forum* 139, no. 1 (1989): 139–167; Kimberle Crenshaw, "Mapping the Margins: Intersectionality, Identity Politics, and Violence Against Women of Color," *Stanford Law Review* 43, no. 6 (1991): 1241–1299.

38. Imogen Tyler, "Resituating Erving Goffman: From Stigma Power to Black Power," *The Sociological Review* 66, no. 4 (2018): 744–765; Imogen Tyler and Tom Slater, "Rethinking the Sociology of Stigma," *The Sociological Review* 66, no. 4 (2018): 721–743.

39. Carmen H. Logie, Llana James, Wangari Tharao, and Mona R. Loutfy, "HIV, Gender, Race, Sexual Orientation, and Sex Work: A Qualitative Study of Intersectional Stigma Experienced by HIV-Positive Women in Ontario, Canada," *PLoS Medicine* 8, no. 11 (2011): e1001124; Carmen Logie, Llana James, Wangari Tharao, and Mona Loutfy, "Associations Between HIV-Related Stigma, Racial Discrimination, Gender Discrimination, and Depression Among HIV-Positive African, Caribbean, and Black Women in Ontario, Canada," *AIDS Patient Care and STDs* 27, no. 2 (2013): 114–122; Valerie A. Earnshaw, Laramie R. Smith, Chinazo O. Cunningham, and Michael M. Copenhaver, "Intersectionality of Internalized HIV Stigma and Internalized Substance Use Stigma: Implications for Depressive Symptoms," *Journal of Health Psychology* 20, no. 8 (2015): 1083–1089; Jenna M. Loyd and Anne Bonds, "Where Do Black Lives Matter? Race, Stigma, and Place in Milwaukee, Wisconsin," *The Sociological Review* 66, no. 4 (2018): 898–918.

40. Carl Latkin, Melissa Davey-Rothwell, Jing-yan Yang, and Natalie Crawford, "The Relationship Between Drug User Stigma and Depression among Inner-City Drug Users in Baltimore, MD," *Journal of Urban Health* 90, no. 1 (2013): 147–156.

41. Mark L. Hatzenbuehler, Jo C. Phelan, and Bruce G. Link, "Stigma as a Fundamental Cause of Population Health Inequalities," *American Journal of Public Health* 103, no. 5 (2013): 813–821. It may also be a driver of socioeconomic inequalities too. See Jo C. Phelan, Jeffrey W. Lucas, Cecilia L. Ridgeway, and Catherine J. Taylor, "Stigma, Status, and Population Health," *Social Science & Medicine* 103 (2014): 15–23.

Conclusion. What We Can Do

1. R. Gardner, "Fatuous and Futile Road to Self-Esteem [Letter to Editor]," *New York Times*, July 30, 1977.

2. Patrick W. Corrigan, Scott B. Morris, Patrick J. Michaels, Jennifer D. Rafacz, and Nicolas Rüsch, "Challenging the Public Stigma of Mental Illness: A Meta-Analysis of Outcome Studies," *Psychiatric Services* 63, no. 10 (2012): 963–973.

3. These leprosy resource materials can be accessed at www.infolep.org/stigma-guides.

4. Laura Nyblade, Anne Stangl, Ellen Weiss, and Kim Ashburn, "Combating HIV Stigma in Health Care Settings: What Works?" *Journal of the International AIDS Society* 12, no. 1 (2009): 15.

5. Sharon Abramowitz, Sarah Lindley McKune, Mosoka Fallah, Josephine Monger, Kodjo Tehoungue, and Patricia A. Omidian, "The Opposite of Denial: Social Learning at the Onset of the Ebola Emergency in Liberia," *Journal of Health Communication* 22, no.1 (2017): 59–65.

6. Sharon Abramowitz, "Ten Things That Anthropologists Can Do to Fight the West African Ebola Epidemic," 2014, http://somatosphere.net/2014/09/ten-things-that-anthropologists-can-do-to-fight-the-west-african-ebola-epidemic.html.

7. Mitchell G. Weiss, Jayashree Ramakrishna, and Daryl Somma, "Health-Related Stigma: Rethinking Concepts and Interventions," *Psychology, Health & Medicine* 11, no. 3 (2006): 277–287.

8. Emily Mendenhall, Kristin Yarris, and Brandon A. Kohrt, "Utilization of Standardized Mental Health Assessments in Anthropological Research: Possibilities and Pitfalls," *Culture, Medicine, and Psychiatry* 40, no. 4 (2016): 726–745.

9. Jonathan M. Metzl and Helena Hansen, "Structural Competency: Theorizing a New Medical Engagement with Stigma and Inequality," *Social Science & Medicine* 103 (2014): 126–133.

10. For an explanation of how this program fits with others, see Paul K. Drain, Charles Mock, David Toole, Anne Rosenwald, Megan Jehn, Thomas Csordas, Laura Ferguson, Caryl Waggett, Chinekwu Obidoa, and Judith N. Wasserheit, "The Emergence of Undergraduate Majors in Global Health: Systematic Review of Programs and Recommendations for Future Directions," *The American Journal of Tropical Medicine and Hygiene* 96, no. 1 (2017): 16–23.

11. A good example of how we are beginning to test this is offered in Jonathan M. Metzl, JuLeigh Petty, and Oluwatunmise V. Olowojoba, "Using a Structural Competency Framework to Teach Structural Racism in Pre-Health Education," *Social Science & Medicine* 199 (2018): 189–201.

12. Jonathan M. Metzl and Helena Hansen, "Structural Competency and Psychiatry," *JAMA Psychiatry* 75, no. 2 (2018): 115–116.

13. Brandon A. Kohrt and Ian Harper, "Navigating Diagnoses: Understanding Mind–Body Relations, Mental Health, and Stigma in Nepal," *Culture, Medicine, and Psychiatry* 32, no. 4 (2008): 462.

14. James L. Griffith and Brandon A. Kohrt, "Managing Stigma Effectively: What Social Psychology and Social Neuroscience Can Teach Us," *Academic Psychiatry* 40, no. 2 (2016): 339–347.

15. Miriam Heijnders and Suzanne Van Der Meij, "The Fight against Stigma: An Overview of Stigma-Reduction Strategies and Interventions," *Psychology, Health & Medicine* 11, no. 3 (2006): 353–363.

16. Danielle M. Raves, Alexandra Brewis, Sarah Trainer, SeungYong Han, and Amber Wutich, "Bariatric Surgery Patients' Perceptions of Weight-Related Stigma in Healthcare Settings Impair Post-Surgery Dietary Adherence," *Frontiers in Psychology* 7 (2016): 1497.

17. N. Rüsch and T. Becker, "Anti-Stigma Interventions in High-and Lower-Income Settings–A Lot Remains to be Done," *Epidemiology and Psychiatric Sciences* 24, no. 5 (2015): 399–401.

18. Lawrence Hsin Yang, Arthur Kleinman, Bruce G. Link, Jo C. Phelan, Sing Lee, and Byron Good, "Culture and Stigma: Adding Moral Experience to Stigma Theory," *Social Science & Medicine* 64, no. 7 (2007): 1524–1535.

19. Loïc Wacquant, *Urban Outcasts: A Comparative Sociology of Advanced Marginality* (Cambridge, UK: Polity Press, 2008).

20. Joan Ablon, "Reflections on Fieldwork with Little People of America: Myths and Methods," in *Others Knowing Others: Perspectives on Ethnographic Careers*, ed. Don D. Fowler and Donald L. Hardesty (Washington, DC: Smithsonian Institution Press, 1994).

21. Joan Ablon, *Little People in America: The Social Dimensions of Dwarfism* (New York: Praeger, 1984). For an historical perspective on Ablon's work, see Russell P. Shuttleworth, "Stigma, Community, Ethnography: Joan Ablon's Contribution to the Anthropology of Impairment-Disability," *Medical Anthropology Quarterly* 18, no. 2 (2004): 139–161.

22. Wacquant, *Urban Outcasts*.

23. Ronald Bayer and Jennifer Stuber, "Tobacco Control, Stigma, and Public Health: Rethinking the Relations," *American Journal of Public Health* 96, no. 1 (2006): 47–50.

24. Farmer has many books and public essays exploring these points. A good place to start is Paul Farmer, *AIDS and Accusation: Haiti and the Geography of Blame*, Updated with a New Preface (Berkeley: University of California Press, 2006).

25. Sarah Trainer, Alexandra Brewis, Amber Wutich, Liza Kurtz, and Monet Niesluchowski, "The Fat Self in Virtual Communities: Success and Failure in Weight-Loss Blogging," *Current Anthropology* 57, no. 4 (2016): 523–528.

26. Testimony by Gary Marx from the Goffman Online Archives at http://cdclv .unlv.edu//ega/.

Appendix

1. Bernice A. Pescosolido and Jack K. Martin, "The Stigma Complex," *Annual Review of Sociology* 41 (2015): 87–116.

2. Erving Goffman, *Stigma: Notes of the Management of Spoiled Identity* (New York: Simon and Shuster, 1963).

3. In this way, "discrimination" is much the same thing as enacted stigma.

4. David L. Vogel, Rachel L. Bitman, Joseph H. Hammer, and Nathaniel G. Wade, "Is Stigma Internalized? The Longitudinal Impact of Public Stigma on Self-Stigma," *Journal of Counseling Psychology* 60, no. 2 (2013): 311.

5. Erika R. Carr, Dawn M. Szymanski, Farah Taha, Lindsey M. West, and Nadine J. Kaslow, "Understanding the Link Between Multiple Oppressions and Depression Among African American Women: The Role of Internalization," *Psychology of Women Quarterly* 38, no. 2 (2014): 233–245.

6. For example, Laura M. Bogart, Burton O. Cowgill, David Kennedy, Gery Ryan, Debra A. Murphy, Jacinta Elijah, and Mark A. Schuster, "HIV-Related Stigma Among People with HIV and Their Families: A Qualitative Analysis," *AIDS and Behavior* 12, no. 2 (2008): 244–254; Joan Ostaszkiewicz, Beverly O'Connell, and Trisha Dunning, "'We Just do the Dirty Work': Dealing with Incontinence, Courtesy Stigma and the Low Occupational Status of Carework in Long-Term Aged Care Facilities," *Journal of Clinical Nursing* 25, no. 17–18 (2016): 2528–2541.

7. Lawrence H. Yang, Fang-pei Chen, Kathleen Janel Sia, Jonathan Lam, Katherine Lam, Hong Ngo, Sing Lee, Arthur Kleinman, and Byron Good, "'What Matters Most': A Cultural Mechanism Moderating Structural Vulnerability and Moral Experience of Mental Illness Stigma," *Social Science & Medicine* 103 (2014): 84–93.

8. Susan Sontag, *AIDS and Its Metaphors*, vol. 1 (New York: Farrar, Straus and Giroux, 1989).

9. Mark L. Hatzenbuehler, "Structural Stigma: Research Evidence and Implications for Psychological Science," *American Psychologist* 71, no. 8 (2016): 742.

10. For example, Alexandra Brewis, Karen L. Schmidt, and Mary Meyer, "ADHD-Type Behavior and Harmful Dysfunction in Childhood: A Cross-Cultural Model," *American Anthropologist* 102, no. 4 (2000): 823–828; Alexandra Brewis and Karen L. Schmidt, "Gender Variation in the Identification of Mexican Children's Psychiatric Symptoms," *Medical Anthropology Quarterly* 17, no. 3 (2003): 376–393.

11. For example, see Amori Yee Mikami, Gua Khee Chong, Jena M. Saporito, and Jennifer Jiwon Na, "Implications of Parental Affiliate Stigma in Families of Children with ADHD," *Journal of Clinical Child & Adolescent Psychology* 44, no. 4 (2015): 595–603.

12. Sarah Trainer, Alexandra Brewis, and Amber Wutich, "Not 'Taking the Easy Way Out': Reframing Bariatric Surgery from Low-Effort Weight Loss to Hard Work," *Anthropology & Medicine* 24, no. 1 (2017): 96–110.

13. For example, Brazilian women with cervical cancer actively perpetuate their shared stigma in ways that reinforce their sense of normalcy and hence support each other. Jessica L. Gregg, "An Unanticipated Source of Hope: Stigma and Cervical Cancer in Brazil," *Medical Anthropology Quarterly* 25, no. 1 (2011): 70–84.

14. S. Kurutz, "Confounding a Smoking Ban, and Bouncers," *New York Times*, August 7, 2013, https://www.nytimes.com/2013/08/08/fashion/smoking-is-back -without-the-stigma.html.

15. Gaylene Becker, "Coping with Stigma: Lifelong Adaptation of Deaf People," *Social Science & Medicine. Part B: Medical Anthropology* 15, no. 1 (1981): 21–24; Carmen H. Logie, LLana James, Wangari Tharao, and Mona R. Loutfy, "HIV, Gender, Race, Sexual Orientation, and Sex Work: A Qualitative Study of Intersectional Stigma Experienced by HIV-Positive Women in Ontario, Canada," *PLoS Medicine* 8, no. 11 (2011): e1001124.

16. Josh Gamson, "Silence, Death, and the Invisible Enemy: AIDS Activism and Social Movement 'Newness,'" *Social Problems* 36, no. 4 (1989): 351–367.

17. Bruce G. Link and Jo C. Phelan, "Conceptualizing Stigma," *Annual Review of Sociology* 27, no. 1 (2001): 363–385.

18. Richard Parker and Peter Aggleton, "HIV and AIDS-Related Stigma and Discrimination: A Conceptual Framework and Implications for Action," *Social Science & Medicine* 57, no. 1 (2003): 13–24.

19. Bruce G. Link and Jo Phelan, "Stigma Power," *Social Science & Medicine* 103 (2014): 24–32.

20. Laura Smart Richman and Micah R. Lattanner, "Self-Regulatory Processes Underlying Structural Stigma and Health," *Social Science & Medicine* 103 (2014): 94–100.

21. Robert Kurzban and Mark R. Leary, "Evolutionary Origins of Stigmatization: The Functions of Social Exclusion," *Psychological Bulletin* 127, no. 2 (2001): 187–208.

22. The number of stable relationships that humans can reasonably maintain seems to be around 150–300. Robin I. M. Dunbar, "Coevolution of Neocortical Size, Group Size and Language in Humans," *Behavioral and Brain Sciences* 16, no. 4 (1993): 681–694; H. Russell Bernard, Gene Ann Shelley, and Peter Killworth, "How Much of a Network Does the GSS and RSW Dredge Up," *Social Networks* 9, no. 1 (1987): 49–61.

23. Patrick W. Corrigan, Jonathon E. Larson, and Nicolas Ruesch, "Self-Stigma and the 'Why Try' Effect: Impact on Life Goals and Evidence-Based Practices," *World Psychiatry* 8, no. 2 (2009): 75–81.

24. Robert M. Sapolsky, "The Influence of Social Hierarchy on Primate Health," *Science* 308, no. 5722 (2005): 648–652; Dickerson, Sally S. Dickerson and Margaret E. Kemeny, "Acute Stressors and Cortisol Responses: A Theoretical Integration and Synthesis of Laboratory Research," *Psychological Bulletin* 130, no. 3 (2004): 355; William W. Dressler, Kathryn S. Oths, and Clarence C. Gravlee, "Race and Ethnicity in Public Health Research: Models to Explain Health Disparities," *Annual Review of Anthropology* 34 (2005): 231–252. For some empirical examples see: Zaneta M. Thayer and Christopher W. Kuzawa, "Ethnic Discrimination Predicts Poor Self-Rated Health and Cortisol in Pregnancy: Insights from New Zealand," *Social Science & Medicine* 128 (2015): 36–42; Heather H. McClure, J. Josh Snodgrass, Charles R. Martinez Jr, J. Mark Eddy, Roberto A. Jiménez, and Laura E. Isiordia, "Discrimination, Psychosocial Stress, and Health Among Latin American Immigrants in Oregon," *American Journal of Human Biology* 22, no. 3 (2010): 421–423.

25. Merrill Singer, Nicola Bulled, Bayla Ostrach, and Emily Mendenhall, "Syndemics and the Biosocial Conception of Health," *The Lancet* 389, no. 10072 (2017): 941–950.

Index

Page numbers in *italics* indicate figures and tables.

About the Authors

Alexandra Brewis and Amber Wutich are both medical anthropologists and President's Professors in the School of Human Evolution and Social Change at Arizona State University, where Alex founded, and Amber now directs, the Center for Global Health. They have five decades of combined experience leading health-relevant field projects globally, including in the Pacific Islands, Australasia, North and South America, Asia, Africa, and the Caribbean. Much of their research has focused on the causes and consequences of people's efforts to cope with two basic, everyday challenges: getting enough safe water and maintaining the "right" body weight.